THE
SURVIVAL RETREAT

THE
SURVIVAL
RETREAT

A TOTAL PLAN FOR RETREAT DEFENSE

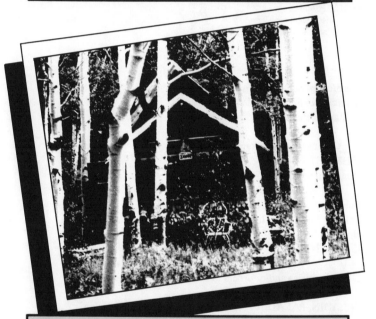

RAGNAR BENSON

PALADIN PRESS
BOULDER, COLORADO

Also by Ragnar Benson:

Acquiring New ID
Breath of the Dragon: Homebuilt Flamethrowers
Bull's-Eye: Crossbows
Do-It-Yourself Medicine
Eating Cheap
Hardcore Poaching
Home-Built Claymore Mines: A Blueprint for Survival
Homemade C-4: A Recipe for Survival
Homemade Grenade Launchers: Constructing the Ultimate Hobby Weapon
Live Off the Land in the City and Country
Mantrapping
Modern Survival Retreat
Modern Weapons Caching
Ragnar's Action Encyclopedias, Volumes 1 and 2
Ragnar's Big Book of Homemade Weapons:
Ragnar's Guide to Home and Recreational Use of High Explosives
Ragnar's Guide to the Underground Economy
Ragnar's Ten Best Traps . . . And a Few Others That Are Damn Good, Too
Survival Poaching
Survivalist's Medicine Chest
Switchblade: The Ace of Blades

The Modern Survival Retreat:
A Total Plan for Retreat Defense
by Ragnar Benson

Copyright © 1983 by Ragnar Benson
ISBN 0-87364-275-9
Printed in the United States of America

Published by Paladin Press, a division of
Paladin Enterprises, Inc., P.O. Box 1307,
Boulder, Colorado 80306, USA.
(303) 443-7250

Direct inquiries and/or orders to the above address.

PALADIN, PALADIN PRESS, and the "horse head" design
are trademarks belonging to Paladin Enterprises and
registered in United States Patent and Trademark Office.

Contents

Introduction

THIS IS NOT ANOTHER BUY-A-main-battle-tank-and-arm-to-the-teeth book about sustaining a three-day firefight with your neighbors after the collapse. My contention is that guns are one of the last, and probably the least important of the major aspects of defending your retreat.

Instead, I have attempted to put together information of genuine practical value that will really teach survivors how to protect their retreats. In doing so, I have drawn heavily on my own experience as well as that of a number of people who have made it through tough, no-holds-barred survival situations. Since no work of this nature could, or should, hold itself out as being the final word, I have also cited quite a lot of current literature.

Survivors with some military background will probably not substantially disagree with my basic retreat defense premises. Conflicts, however, will arise when this material is compared with the theories of those quasi survivalists whose volumes of writing often vastly exceeds their on-the-ground experience. I suspect that the main reason some of these people have so many followers is because many Americans want a good excuse to buy a lot of guns. Some of the armament gurus

1

will gladly justify purchasing a whole roomful of firearms!

However, survival, and especially retreat defense, is a personal matter. It is not something that can be decided on for you by your neighbors, your friends, your priest, survivalist writers like myself, or the government. All that experts like myself can do is offer suggestions, hopefully based on good, solid experience. You, the survivor, will have to be the final judge of that.

Because retreat defense is an individual matter, I feel you should acquire as much on-the-ground experience as you can. When you do, it will become painfully obvious that some of the gurus don't have as much experience as you thought they did. With some field experience behind you, you will find it infinitely easier to develop and implement your own plan.

In late December 1967, I was traveling with a small private military outfit hired by a central African government that has long since dropped into the bottomless pit of oblivion. Our raiding party—that's all it really was—consisted of eleven dirty, grungy, godforsaken Europeans mounted on three Rovers, one pulling a trailer with gear and ammo, one with a mounted .50 caliber machine gun, and the third with a socket and tire setup for a small clip-fed .30. One of our guys was a third generation Kenyan who had first fought as a teenager during the Mau Mau Rebellion. The entire crew was hard-core refuse, swept up in the maelstrom of dirty little African wars that no one has ever heard of.

We were on the road for six days. Much of that time was spent fooling around doing nothing while we lulled the bush telegraph into indifference. Some days our little column made but thirty or so kilometers when we could easily have done eighty. But our leisurely pace and deliberately circuitous route precluded that.

Around noon on the fifth day we pulled up early and camped off the road in a small, obscure wash about forty-five kilometers from our target village. The men spent the afternoon sleeping and cleaning their weapons.

Shortly after dark, the eleven of us pulled out again, now heading directly for our assigned target. Our mission was to hit a village of about ten thousand souls a few kilometers across an ill-defined border. The village had been the source and refuge of some antigovernment terrorists, and the central authorities for whom we were working had decided that it was time to "give some instruction in foreign policy." As the only "unofficial" member of the group, I had a rare opportunity to see how foreign policy is practiced in some of the less developed nations.

Seven kilometers north of the village our column split into two groups. Another fellow and I headed southwest on foot; the rest drove northwest on the road across the high savannah. Recent burning had cleared most of the tangle; we had a relatively pleasant walk in the cool, damp moonlight.

Just before first light, we reached our assigned position on a gentle rise about twenty meters above and eighty meters to the side of the dusty, rutted road leading to the village. Our instructions were to place ourselves about one to one and a half kilometers out. Since neither of us had ever been in the area before, we could only guess at our exact location. The village was not in sight, although we could hear cattle now and then. The wind was wrong to smell it.

As the sky grew lighter, I could make out about twelve Hunter's hartebeest moving across a grassy flat upwind of us. They moved hesitantly, taking a little nip of new grass now and then. As soon as I could see well enough, I picked out a nice young buck and dropped him with one shot from my Browning .338. The noise of the pistol shot echoed through the gentle hills. My companion was so startled, he fell off the termite nest on which he had been sitting.

According to the instructions we had been given, we were supposed to shoot the first villager who happened along the road that morning. As it worked out, the hartebeest was a better choice. There was plenty of bloodshed a bit later without our adding anything to it. As an extra benefit, we enjoyed fresh meat that afternoon for the first time in six days.

I set to work gutting the critter and was almost done when the other group's guns opened up. The plan had called for the two of us to create a diversion that would scare the villagers out to the other side of town into range of the machine guns. Apparently my one shot had put the plan in motion. We could hear the steady purr of the .30 along with the metered fire of the FNs. Over all that, the giant .50 caliber thump-thump-thumped regularly. After about five minutes the shooting subsided. We walked cautiously on up toward the village on the dusty little road. Had we even supposed that anyone had anything more than a gas pipe gun, it would have been an act of incredible bravado.

In those days the flow of Soviet weapons into the region had not yet reached flood stage. I felt safe enough, but a kind of sick self-consciousness made me want to melt into the stinking, dry village dirt as we passed through. Most of the villagers had fled. A few women and children, old men, and a cripple or two were all that remained. Those who couldn't run away watched us pass with horribly scared white eyes from behind the boonahs and randaavels. The few shops were all deserted.

The scene on the other side of town was horrible,

the more so for the presence of the remains of the one hundred fifty or so cows that had been caught in the ambush. The only redeeming factor I could think of was that, in their rush to escape, the men had abandoned their women and children. They had tried to save only their most precious possessions and their own lives, which was why so many cows got it. Women in Africa are treated worse than cattle. The upside of the ambush was that, in comparison to the men, very few women got hurt. Usually it's the other way around.

There are four valuable lessons in this story for the retreat defender. The first is don't ever become a target for those who can hurt you. Be inconspicuous and stay out of sight. The wise survivor does not become a lesson in foreign policy.

The second is that no matter how well armed you are and how hardened your retreat, you can't hold out even briefly against a well-trained, well-armed military force. We knew that some of the African villagers had weapons and were fairly proficient with them; yet they were spooked and overrun in minutes.

The third lesson may be obscure at this point: it is don't ever become a refugee. Stake out your home turf and stay there, defending it as best you can.

Fourth and last, we should never have been able to walk through that village after the shooting. You should *never* give up your ability or desire to resist. This assumes that you have both the equipment and the desire to begin with. In the case of the African village, the outcome would have been the same; it just wouldn't have been so damn easy. A psychological element of retreat defense is forfeited when the defenders are known to possess neither the means nor the will to fight.

As I said at the beginning, a lot of things are more

important than guns. In this example, we could list things like regular patrols, sentries, a plan of resistance, a basic defense network, rules against openly and notoriously harboring terrorists, and a set of values based on something more precious than cows.

Each element has its place in a viable retreat defense strategy, and each is, in its way, as important as guns. The important point is that defenders should understand the rules and then set out to play the game wisely and with determination. To that end, I dedicate this book to those who are willing to defend their retreats no matter what the cost—*even if it means staying out of a firefight.*

1. Why Retreat?

W HY RETREAT?" IS A QUESTION that 90 percent of our population cannot and will not answer. If they could, that same 90 percent of our friends, neighbors, and countrymen would have to admit that things may not continue on as they are now. They would also have to admit that they will need a retreat—something completely impossible for the average American to do.

Certainly part of the problem lies with the hopelessly pessimistic attitude the peacemongers have encouraged. According to several national polls, a minimum of 80 percent of us genuinely believe that no one will survive a general nuclear attack. These people have given up already.

I certainly plan to make it through a nuclear attack, and I sincerely believe you can make it through as well. If you doubt this, try reading Bruce Clayton's excellent book *Life After Doomsday* (see bibliography). It will do more to instill spirit and hope than anything else I can think of. Other worthwhile reading is the editorial series run by the *Wall Street Journal* in early 1982. The *Journal* did an extremely credible job of tracing the antinuke peace movement's leadership back to the Kremlin and of documenting the fact that the Soviets genuinely believe they can emerge victorious from a nuclear confrontation. The *Journal*'s material closely parallels my own experience and coincides with what my mother, who was Russian, taught me about dealing with the Soviets.

Besides the nuclear threat, there is also the very real possibility of economic collapse or social breakdown, either of which would sweep away most restraints that we take for granted in our society. The French political philosopher Frederic Bastiat pointed out that governments that promise things to their people end up disappointing most of them when the politicians can't really deliver on those promises. In other words, the more promises a government makes, the shakier it becomes. The end result is either anarchy or a dictatorship.

At this writing, unemployment is at a forty-year, 11 percent high. Still, Americans call upon the government to "do something." I'll leave it up to the reader to decide if the greater danger lies in nuclear confrontation or in governmental breakdown.

As I said earlier, the first step in preparing to survive is to admit that some kind of collapse will eventually occur and that during that time you, your family, and your friends will need a suitable place to hole up. Having made, what for many is an incredibly tough decision, you must also settle two more issues before embarking on a program to build your retreat.

For the purposes of this book and for your survival in general, I will not agree that you really believe you can and will survive, unless a plan of action accompanies that belief. In other words, *you must believe enough to start doing something,* and that something must be based on a credible, realistic plan.

The next step—one I have faced many times over

starting when I was a young man in Cuba on my first international assignment—is to evaluate accurately and calmly what sort of danger you will actually be facing. This step is so important that I have written an entire chapter on the subject. What one must know here is not who, but in a broad sense, what. Is it chemical warfare, pestilence, nuclear warfare, famine, an occupying army, earthquakes, floods, or rioting plunderers? To simplify matters let me say that the basic defense concepts are pretty much the same no matter what the threat. The only things that really change are the defense tools you stockpile in your retreat. These can vary, depending on what it is that seems likely to get you. Basic strategies, however, remain unchanged for the most part.

For instance, I feel that the danger of our government attempting to suppress American guerrilla fighters in rural areas of our country is very real. The Soviets have said over and over that they intend to strike first at our military bases; having destroyed our ability to retaliate to any meaningful degree, they will then threaten to destroy twenty or thirty large cities if we don't surrender. Given the records of most of our politicians, I believe we will, as a country, capitulate. When there is nobody other than the victims around to complain, the Soviet record is consistent—witness Laos, Cambodia, Vietnam, and Afghanistan. They will move in using gas and chemicals to liquidate people and poison farmlands. For this reason I keep decontamination suits and filter breathing apparatus in my retreat, something I would not do if all I expected to face were looters rioting after their food stamps were cut off.

Setting up a retreat is, for the most part, practicing the art of the possible. It's a matter of wisely and shrewdly identifying what you have available and turning it into something usable. People who can do this easily and well we describe as having *street sense*. Street sense is acquired through experiencing adversity and desperation. Those who have street sense have a tremendous advantage over those who have never had to go out and "scratch shit with the chickens."

About three years ago the editor of one of the major gun magazines mentioned to me that she appreciated a magazine article I wrote on urban survival. Up to that time, she said, she had always assumed that "everyone living in places like New York, Chicago, or Los Angeles was simply going to die." The only way she could expect to survive was to leave New York—something she could not do then and something she felt would be "impossible later, after the collapse."

Many urban survivors believe that they must evacuate to a rural retreat to make it. Having lived in both environments and having watched several mini-collapses in Africa and the Middle and Far East, I know this is not true. People who are not rural by nature and upbringing should stay away from farms. They simply will not make it in a tightly knit agricultural environment. If you have street sense rather than field sense, stay on the streets. People survive in cities and you can, too, especially in the U.S. where food is currently cheap and can be stockpiled without much difficulty or expense.

Current civil defense thinking envisions turning our entire nation into a mob of refugees. Lacking an adequate shelter system, the program calls for evacuating the cities and sending everyone out into the country to live until the bombing is over. For survivors who either live in the country or would be pushed out of the city, a number of red flags should go up. Where will all these millions of people go? What will they eat? Whose toilet will they flush? Whose property will they flood over onto? How will they be moved? All are perfectly valid questions which have, of course, no rational answers.

STAYING PUT

As a general rule the survivor is better off staying on his home ground and building his retreat there. Rational evacuation plans have their place, but in general the survivor will find it easier to plan, stock, move to, and defend a retreat that is either in his home or at least located in his home territory.

In my book *Eating Cheap* (see bibliography), I devoted a chapter to the art of doing business with rural people. I have found that farmers are so different in their ways of thinking and acting that unless you have prior experience in dealing with these people, it is absolute idiocy to leave the city in an emergency and expect to coexist with them. You will be dead and gone within a month if you try it.

There are some exceptions. Wealthy people who have built rural retreats or members of survival units who have established safe areas in the country are two examples. However, remember that these people are not refugees; they have well-thought-through evacuation plans which they can implement when the time comes. The fact that these plans call for them to move to the country has nothing to do with my original warning. They will not become refugees.

But getting back to the two important questions I alluded to earlier, the first point one must consider is, "Where will I stay during and after the collapse?" It is absolutely essential that survivors have a clear, concise, well-thought-through plan that is perfectly plausible to implement the moment a national or regional crisis occurs that honestly, practically addresses this issue.

REFUGEES

As I implied in my introduction, there is nothing more tragic and more pitiful than a refugee. Refugees are people without hope who have left their homes to run ahead of the holocaust, never in control of their own destinies. They are people who must rely on the charity of others until their time runs out and they die. I have seen them in Sudan and in the Northern Frontier District of Kenya, in northern Somalia, Ethiopia, Jordan and Lebanon, on the southeast coast of Florida, and in scores of other places throughout the world. All of these people have one thing in common: utter hopelessness.

The important lesson you can learn from this book is *never,* under any circumstances, ever become a refugee. Evaluate your situation and circumstances. Make your plan and then, by God, win, lose, or draw—even when its weaknesses start to show up—stick with your prearranged scenario. Be flexible, versatile, and sensitive to what's happening; but most of all, implement your plan and basically stick with it. Die if you must, but die on your home turf with your face to the wind, not in some stinking hellhole 2,000 kilometers away, among people you neither know nor care about.

I was marginally involved when Saigon fell to the North Vietnamese. I would have had a tougher time if I hadn't befriended an Agency employee who had a good idea what was coming and had meticulously planned out three separate, workable evacuation routes. Each made use of completely different modes of transportation and did not depend on the success of the other two. When the time came, he put the best plan under the circumstances in motion, and we got out.

Even more than defending a retreat, getting to a safe area requires a great deal of skill. This guy was, among other things, a helicopter pilot, a seasoned paratrooper, a good boat captain, a jogger, a motorcycle operator, and a long-distance patrol leader. All survivalists must be versatile with strong skills in a number of areas. Yet this fellow amazed even me. Because the subject of getting to one's retreat is so important, I have devoted an entire chapter to this subject.

2. What Is a Retreat?

A RETREAT IS A PLACE WHERE you will find the shelter and protection, food and water, medicine and warmth you prepared for yourself until society returns to its normal, nondestructive, repetitious rut. Sometimes the eventual "stabilization" leaves something to be desired, but even in places like Iran, Cambodia, and Chile, some sort of normalcy eventually returns.

Usually this takes about two years. There is first a period of intense dislocation, lasting perhaps six months. This is followed by a time of reaping, when things don't necessarily get worse but people continue to die by the thousands as a result of what has previously occurred. This stage is somewhat like the crash in deer and rabbit populations: as soon as the numbers are down, the situation stabilizes.

The trick here is to have a retreat prepared wherein you can be one of the survivors. Your retreat can be in the city, in the country, where you work, or at a close friend's or relative's place. The important point is that your retreat is a place where you go to live through the crisis, and not a hole you crawl into to die.

A retreat must be out of the mainstream of looting and burning or be camouflaged and fireproofed to escape these hazards. Since there is a great likelihood of nuclear, biological, or chemical warfare, a retreat must protect from these dangers as well. It has to be stocked with food, fuel, and clothing and contain the core means with which to start a new life after the collapse and resulting dislocations.

I know scores of people who have set up their retreats in the basements of their houses. Others have apartments in large concrete buildings that will probably do almost as nicely. A farmer I know plans to use a root cellar on his land . . . after dynamiting the two road bridges leading across the creeks onto his property. Another man intends to pull a self-contained travel camper into an underground parking garage near his home.

A group in Washington State plans to establish a tent camp in a sheltered valley along a small river, while the inhabitants of a small community in southern Utah intend to live pretty much as they do now—except that all contact with the outside world will be severed. They plan to work together to be completely self-reliant. Their only requirement is that all members must be Mormon and must do their share of work. These people are rough on folks with a welfare mentality.

In suburbia I have seen garages and recreation rooms outfitted with extra-strong walls and roofs, filtered ventilation systems, and food and water supplies that will support the inhabitants for months or even years. Shop buildings are another common retreat location. With a bit of prior planning and work, these types of buildings can be made into outstanding retreats.

The important point is that survivors who will occupy these retreats have turned off their tubes and put some thought into evaluating possible dangers and what they will need to do to survive. I have a close friend who claims that a retreat is 90 percent psycholo-

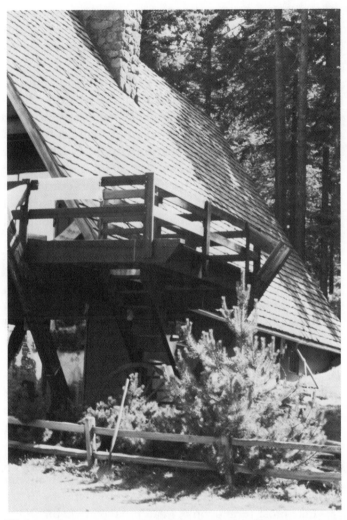

This home also serves as a survivalist's retreat. It was built with twelve-inch concrete walls in the basement and butted into the side of a hill. Trees provide camouflage and fuel for cooking and heating via the fireplace.

gical; perhaps he is right. Some retreats are so simple that they are nothing more than a hole in the backyard. What makes them a retreat per se is the will and determination of the owner.

I myself have almost always lived in the country. My retreat is in my home, built over a large, sturdy basement into the side of a mountain. In many ways it is the classic "desert island" hideaway that many survivalists fantasize about. The foundation has thirty-centimeter walls and is dug into three meters of solid earth. Three stories above provide distance and mass protection against nuclear dangers. I have my own well, a diesel generator, four years' supply of food, medical supplies, abundant guns and ammo, a large garden spot, stored seeds, fuel oil, chemicals and fertilizer, decontamination and breathing gear, explosives, and so on.

This may seem ideal, but am I really better off than the city dweller who has reinforced a basement in a concrete building? He might have to store a bit more food than I do, but even after the collapse he will have better access to manufactured goods. In many respects, his retreat will be more secure. I suspect that bands of scavengers will be scouring the country looking for places like mine. Even in remote areas like mine, there will be many ugly situations as looters attempt to gain their means of survival by force. Furthermore, the city survivor will be in or near his retreat when the time comes. I may have a struggle just getting to my retreat if I am traveling, as is often the case.

Like most rural people, I can't make my living in the country. I will probably be working in a large city when the collapse occurs. Perhaps I will have some warning and will be able to take off with the two extra cans of gas that I always keep in the car. Perhaps not. There is always my airplane, which I keep near—but will I be able to fly it? My last-ditch plan to buy or steal a motorcycle may not even be viable. Only time will tell.

Even more than my domestic plans to reach my retreat, I am concerned about the number of foreign assignments I have recently received. In time of crisis, how will I get back from the Philippines, Sudan, India, or even southern Mexico?

The city dweller has fewer of these worries. As Bruce Clayton points out, the dangers of nuclear attack are greatly exaggerated. The most serious dangers will be much the same for the country dweller. In *Live Off the Land in the City and Country* (see bibliography), I recommend that the city dweller stockpile twice as much food and water. The plan for the urban survivor involves total seclusion for months on end until it is safe to come out. Then you can barter your skills and the hardware available in the city with rural people who will be coming to town for items they can't make.

The dieback will have occurred. Your retreat will have served its purpose, and it will be time to start building a new economy.

As I have pointed out, a retreat is a place you go to live. Not die. It is a place out of the mainstream of events that contains the means to survive without outside support. It is defensible and is put together with a realistic understanding of what the dangers will be. It is both a plan and an inventory.

Building the retreat itself is almost always anticlimactic. The hardest part is admitting you need a retreat and then putting together a plan. It's like the country of Switzerland: the mountains constitute a mighty fortress, but as the Swiss admit, one must know how to man the fortress and be willing to do so when the time comes. I trust this chapter will break the impasse for you and that you will get on with the work at hand.

3. Practical Retreat Designs

No MATTER HOW YOU CUT IT, the best, most practical retreats are those built underground.

This is not to say that aboveground retreats can't be put together. Some have worked admirably well for long periods of time, especially in larger cities. But it is easier, cheaper, and better to go underground, especially if you must plan for the full spectrum of problems. Retreats, for instance, should be reasonably airtight. Constant temperature control is important, as is fire resistance. As a means of protection against nuclear blast forces, underground shelters are almost ideal. Anything else is a lot more trouble.

One of the best books on retreat construction is *Improvised Fallout Shelters in Buildings,* published in August 1972 by the University of Idaho College of Engineering. Its information pertains to using existing buildings, from grain bins to old stores, for retreats. Virtually the only situations the authors endorse are basements. The Office of Civil Defense also has several publications on retreat construction; all but one of these are for underground designs. These include *Family Home Shelter Designs* (PSD F-61-1), *Home Shelter* (H-12-1), and *Aboveground Home Shelter.* One of the tricks I was

21

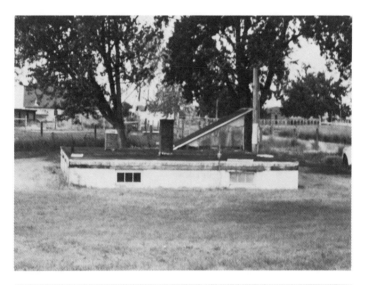

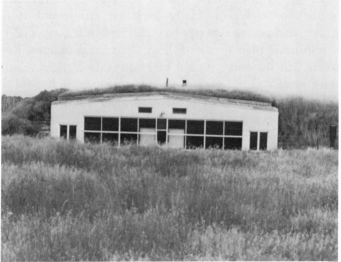

Underground houses like the one on top can be very useful as shelters.
However, they aren't much fun to live in. The underground house on the
bottom is camouflaged from three sides, gives good earthen protection, and
yet allows good light and ventilation.

reminded of in these pamphlets was the extensive use of sandbags. Perhaps the more correct name should be cloth bags filled with earth. Ex-military people will remember spending hours filling and stacking sandbags to form bunkers and gun emplacements. Retreaters will likely find themselves doing the same thing the first weeks after the collapse.

Explosion-proof structures must be *ductile;* meaning they have to give and spring back. A deep basement with a sandbag-reinforced first floor is ideal under these circumstances, but one item that is not stressed enough in any of the publications I have seen is the absolutely vital need to reinforce the floor heavily over any basement retreat. I recommend putting up twice as many supports as seem necessary, then doubling that. In 1968 I saw some buildings in the Gaza Strip that were heavily damaged, but the combination of sandbagging and reinforcement kept even heavy mortar rounds from doing much damage to the people sheltered below. Standard steel floor joist jacks are available at lumberyards. Retreaters should buy them now or at least lay in materials with which to construct floor supports. Another thing I will do if I have enough warning is to fill a couple of water beds on the first floor over my basement retreat. The stored water will be useful and in case of fire may provide effective protection for us and our supplies. In addition, water acts as a modest barrier against gamma rays.

My favorite retreat design when building from scratch is basically a modified root cellar. The best source of information on root cellars that I have seen is *Stocking Up* (see bibliography).

ROOT CELLARS

A root cellar is fairly easy to build using unskilled

labor, and even an elaborate model is relatively cheap. A further advantage is that a root cellar can be built in stages. The unfinished product won't be very comfortable if it must be occupied before completion, but it will provide most of the needed protection, and it will sustain life. In the interim, a root cellar makes a great place to store food.

Root cellars require very little space and can be put in most backyards. The traditional models used by farmers and ranchers for centuries aren't big enough to be retreats, but minor increases in size can be made at very little expense. Root cellars require a small piece of well-drained property on which to be built. For many city survivors, especially those living in high rises, this may seem unlikely, but things change and unusual opportunities sometimes come up.

The basic difference between a conventional root cellar and a retreat is the ventilation system, size, depth in the ground, roof reinforcement, and some work on the approaches to the area where the cellar is located.

Ventilation first. Since the total enclosed area of a cellar retreat is extremely limited (compared to one built in a larger basement or on the ninth floor of a concrete high rise), the survivor will have to install a filtered ventilation system. My basement retreat is dug three meters deep into the side of a mountain, and three stories cover the shelter. I won't need a forced air ventilation system because the space has breathing room and is somewhat filtered by the mass above. For a conventional, below-ground root cellar, the simple hand-operated ventilation system outlined in *Nuclear War Survival Skills* (see bibliography) can be built with eight meters of plastic pipe, a cover, and a pull flap.

Obscure the ventilation outlet. The best I have seen was located twenty meters from the cellar and looked

Ventilation System for Root Cellar Retreat

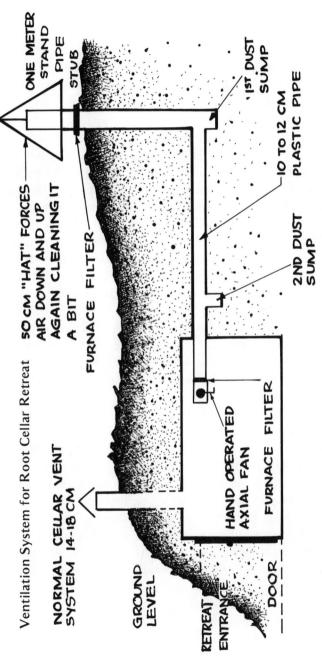

ONE METER STAND PIPE

STUB

50 CM "HAT" FORCES AIR DOWN AND UP AGAIN CLEANING IT A BIT

FURNACE FILTER

1ST DUST SUMP

10 TO 12 CM PLASTIC PIPE

2ND DUST SUMP

NORMAL CELLAR VENT SYSTEM 14-18 CM

HAND OPERATED AXIAL FAN

FURNACE FILTER

RETREAT ENTRANCE

GROUND LEVEL

DOOR

Drawing air into the retreat through a ventilation system creates a positive air pressure that tends to keep dust from seeping in. Natural warm air ventilation may be sufficient for the retreat if there are few people and filters are not placed in the line.

like part of an underground lawn sprinkler system.

Dig your cellar deep into a hill, if possible. If not, put it deep into the ground with just a narrow little stairway leading down to the door. The roof should have at least *one* meter of earth covering it. The cellar should be no less than two meters deep and four meters long. The width can be as narrow as two meters, but three is better. By building the cellar four meters long and two meters wide, two bunks can be built end to end stacked three deep. The beauty of a deep cellar is that it will be better insulated and self-regulated for both heat and cold, and afford better protection from NBC threats. The cellar's temperature stays at a constant 15 degrees centigrade to 18 degrees centigrade year round, unless it is packed with people.

Water is important. Make certain that the site you pick is well drained. On the other hand, you will also need a water source for domestic use. As you develop and improve your retreat, you may want to install water and fuel oil tanks, or drill a well in the floor of the cellar if that's possible.

A cellar can initially be built with scrounged material and hard work. A healthy male could dig the hole in most places in two weekends. Initially the floor can be gravel or clay, although eventually it should be concreted. In many soils the walls can be left bare at first, or if necessary be made out of treated rough-cut lumber. The roof can be constructed of rough planks supported by posts, although a cement roof slab held up by steel posts is better. It takes three times as many wooden posts to hold up a rough earthen roof, which restricts your movement in the shelter. All of the cement work can be done in small sections by the survivalist himself for very little money. We are talking about a maximum of eighteen cubic meters of concrete.

Hand mixed, the cost would not exceed $360!

The door and approaches are important on any retreat. The entrance should be sheltered from fallout and provide a cleanup place for those coming and going. It won't do to drag "yellow rain" into your retreat on your boots. Almost all commercial and governmental retreat designs fail to address this necessary consideration. Eventually you will have to spend some money on the doors to your retreat. Beg, borrow, or steal some heavy, massive steel commercial doors if possible. Make sure they fit tightly, If you have space to put in double doors, do so, including a firing port in the first door.

In terms of security, hopefully your neighbors will think it quaint that you are building a root cellar and soon forget about it. You may want to build a rock garden or something similar around your area to be reinforced later with sandbags as a slit trench system. It isn't a good idea to operate this close to the actual retreat, but you may have to use these trenches as a last-ditch defense area.

It may be possible to prevent a mob from getting into your cellar, but regular police and military forces will not have much trouble once they get on top of your roof. That's why the perimeter defense mechanisms mentioned in later chapters are so important.

BASEMENT SHELTERS

People with small lots in the city may want to cement-block off a corner of a basement to accomplish basically the same objective as the root cellar. In this case, the shelter is a kind of box in a box. Again, be sure to brace up the ceiling adequately, provide for fire protection, put in a good, solid door and fill the masonry blocks with concrete. After you are done, pile junk

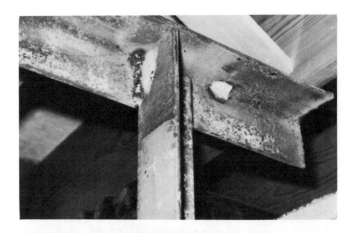

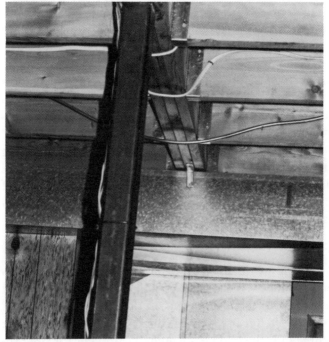

These devices for reinforcing the basement ceiling were homemade from angle iron. Note the twelve-inch interior supporting wall in the center of the bottom photo.

around the walled-in corner to camouflage the structure
and make it hard to get to.

HIGH-RISE SHELTERS

The same thing can be done on the upper levels of
a high rise. If you are on an upper floor in an apartment
complex and intend to stay there, be sure to provide
additional roof bracing, or you may well get caved in
on. In my climate, heating and cooling can also be a
problem. And remember that underground retreats provide much better protection from NBC threats.

IMPROVISED SHELTERS

Road tunnels, public building basements, subway
tunnels, and bridge underpasses are all possibilities. Although their public nature makes them tough to secure
and develop, don't completely overlook them. Old
boilers, coal storage areas, fuel tanks, stores (with basements), old mines, quarries, and potato cellars are other
good places to develop retreats.

There are a lot of plans kicking around for tempo-
rary shelters dug, foxhole style, into a hill, or made in
boats or on land with car bodies. I strongly suspect that
most of the people who use these will not survive; there
is no defense plan that can be implemented, no food
and water, and little protection from the elements,
much less the NBC hazards or the howling mobs. I don't
believe as a practical matter they will work. By implica-
tion, there is no prior planning to this type of shelter
and, as I said earlier, people without plans are not going
to be survivors.

Whatever else you do, don't let yourself be herded
into a common underground shelter with masses of
people who have made no preparations. If you do, you
will be deprived of your guns and ammo, your food,

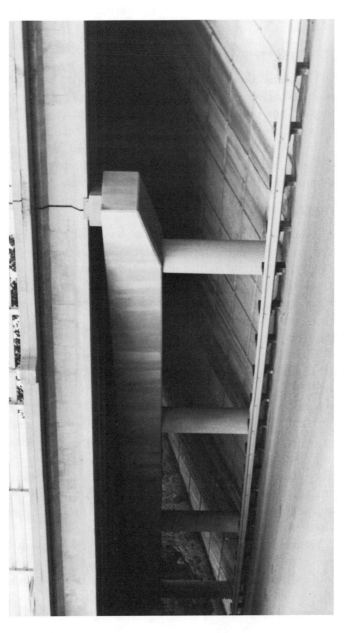

You might decide to blow up a bridge such as this in order to limit traffic to your retreat. Or if you haven't planned far enough ahead to have prepared a retreat, you might be able to use the nooks and crannies of a bridge like this one for shelter.

your liberty, your sophisticated survival equipment and, worst of all, your control over your own destiny!

About the best plan I have seen is the one that is being put together by the Mormon Church, mostly in the central West. The plan has many elements; and, given the Mormons' propensity to use force, including lethal force, on outsiders, may not be the best for others living around the area. It will, nevertheless, be advantageous for the Mormons and of interest to other survivors.

In the rural areas they dominate, the Mormons plan to function as complete, integrated communities, cut off from the rest of the world much as they do now. Where the Mormons do not dominate, but where their numbers are many, they have begun developing "Mormon Bunkers." These are large, extremely well-built homes on ample, readily tillable plots of land situated in places that can be easily defended. Usually a wealthy doctor or dentist will make the initial land purchase. The building will be constructed using volunteer labor organized by the church on a piece-by-piece basis. The bunkers I have seen have huge, deep basements, two wells, large water storage capacity, 12,000 liter fuel oil storage, generators, bunkrooms and incredible food supplies. There are garden tools, freezers, barns for livestock, shooting ranges, guard dogs, canning facilities, and much more. I have a friend who lives within a kilometer of one of these places. He says that all of the Mormons in the area will collect at the bunker after the collapse.

The possibly fatal flaw in this plan is that the houses are so large and conspicuous that they attract attention. Even though almost all are a ways out of town, they may well wind up under constant siege by desperate people seeking food and refuge.

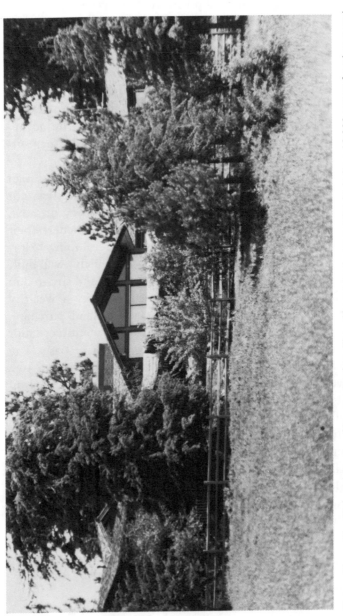

Pictured is a self-sufficient retreat—a Mormon bunker. The self-contained community includes a 10,000-square-foot house and numerous outbuildings. In case of crisis, communications with the outside world would come to an abrupt halt.

The actual retreat must rely on the art of the practical. You will, to a large extent, have to use what is available. Invariably, clever people can put something together. Survivors will be clever people.

4. What Do You Have to Protect?

R ETREATS CAN EASILY BECOME
the targets of hostile enemy force, but not for the reasons many people think. I saw this several times in Africa. Our retreats were attacked, not because they were sound, comfortable shelters well-stocked with essential goods, but because they were symbols of resistance and defiance that might, as a bonus, contain items worth plundering.

This brings us to the question: What do you have to protect? The answer, of course, is virtually everything needed to keep body and soul together. The point is that attackers sometimes don't want your supplies; what they do want is to destroy the independence your supplies afford you. The desperate starving horde isn't always your chief problem.

CACHES

In *Live Off the Land in the City and Country,* I explained my caching strategy. One important element of that strategy involves burying several 20-centimeter waterproof tubes containing basic supplies of food, medicine, guns, and ammo. A very simple basic stock of these items might prove to be invaluable should you lose your retreat by occupation, disaster, or other causes.

The supplies I have cached in tubes around the country can only provide a makeshift existence. Unlike more than 90 percent of the people planning to survive the holocaust, I have actually had some experience living this way, and it's a miserable, precarious existence. If I am uncertain whether I can make it, what chance has the deskbound city dweller of living a hand-to-mouth existence out of the limited supplies in his cache? The answer is that caching is only a stopgap measure. Almost all of what it will take to survive must be contained in one's retreat. It's like a rocket ship hurtling through space—there is no way to go back and resupply; everything required for life must be there, not necessarily in luxurious abundance, but it must be there.

Before talking about how to prioritize your needs, there is one other point that I want to bring up. When planning for the post-collapse economy, the survivor must accurately assess the status of property rights in his home area. In Watts a few years back, and in Newark, Miami, and London, fairly minor incidents triggered widespread rioting, burning, and looting. In many cases the rioters burned down the very buildings they lived in! By contrast, in Poland, in rural America in the Depression years, and in Turkey at the close of their period of anarchy in late 1979, a lot of truly grim things happened, but people did not plunder the goods of their fellow citizens, nor did they burn their own homes. The difference, I think, was due to a widely held respect for individual property rights. Even the Poles, who supposedly live in a propertyless, Communist state, still seem to retain many of the values of private ownership.

People do not destroy property that belongs to someone. They destroy property that belongs to "no one," such as government-owned inner-city property, or for that matter the federal forest lands that have been raped by timber companies and vacationers alike.

If your retreat is located in the inner city, where the idea of private property has been obsolete for a good many years, watch out. Your neighbors will believe that what is yours can be theirs simply because the idea of ownership is incomprehensible. If those around you know you intend to resist, the problem may be magnified. The best protection is to be in an out-of-the-way place, unobtrusive, hardened to the dangers ahead, and completely invisible to others. Avoid becoming a target or *cause celèbre* at all cost.

If what you have to protect is what it takes to stay alive, then it is important to list those items. Staying alive, after all, is your major concern.

FOOD AND WATER

The first, most important need that people must satisfy is for water and food. Some years back, I wrote a magazine article on the necessity of planning for a source of water. I made a list of things like equipment for driving and pumping your own well, water collection devices, water desalination and purification equipment, suggested places to find water especially in the city, and an interim water storage program. No one would publish it then, something that is certainly not true today.

Your food supply is vitally important. I suggest approaching it in two ways—food you can store and items such as fertilizer, insecticides, tools, garden seeds, and traps that you can store to produce food. As part of a production program, you should also develop some means of extending your food's shelf life. In the Philippines I have seen potatoes go from twelve cents a kilo to one dollar in a week because the farmers had no way of successfully storing their produce.

SHELTER

After food and water, the next need is shelter. Make sure your shelter will, in fact, protect you from the likely dangers. Does it need to be fireproof, bombproof, chemical/biological proof? If it does, then put it together that way.

I live 300 kilometers downwind from a SAC base. I expect to face a couple of weeks of fairly intense nuclear fallout. To mitigate this danger, I dug our basement into the side of a mountain, built the foundation 30 cm. thick and constructed three stories over the basement to put some distance between the fallout and me. I also cast thirty-eight lead sheets 8 cm. x 16 cm. x 3 cm. thick to use over our bunk beds as additional shielding. I've also laid in survey meters, dosimeters, air filtration devices, and personal decontamination suits.

Another necessary component of a retreat that is virtually always overlooked is heat. Easily implemented plans can be made to stay warm and can include everything from issuing two sweaters to everyone to installing an oil-fired central heating system.

MEDICINE

The retreat must have adequate medical supplies. I addressed this subject in the *Survivalist's Medicine Chest* (see bibliography) and Bruce Clayton covered it nicely in *Life After Doomsday*. I recommend that you stock medications and equipment to the absolute maximum level of your medical competence. Be sure to include a good survival library of many good books containing hardcore practical information. Medical books come to mind first, but there are many others covering everything from gardening to firearms repair and modification.

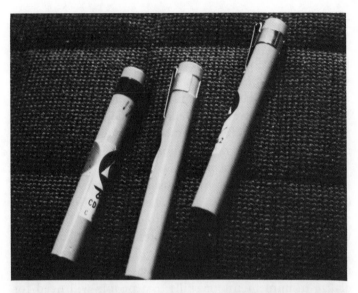

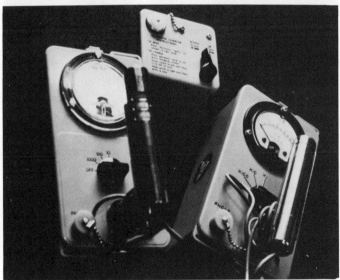

Individual dosimeters (top) are worn on the belt and are essential for counting the radioactivity each member of a group is exposed to. Survey meters (bottom) count the radioactivity in an area. Note the dosimeter charger pictured between the two survey meters.

TOOLS

Other necessities are tools and supplies with which to make your living in the post-collapse economy. You will need carpentry tools, gunsmithing and reloading equipment, agricultural implements, and many others. Don't forget that even the native Indians specialized in producing their wares and that you will, too, if you are going to fit into the next economy.

For the same reason, I have laid in an extensive line of barter goods. Any irresponsible government official can smear ink on paper and call it money. Items of real worth will be items with day-to-day value. It is very, very easy to lay in the wrong barter goods, especially for those who are currently getting their experience in the underground economy, so plan wisely. Choose to specialize in implements or skills that people will need for their survival. Remember the value of the blacksmith, shoe cobbler, tinsmith, and tailor?

Clothing is something that seems more important than it really is. Most people in a survival situation will have enough to wear. If nothing else, clothes can be scrounged from the dead.

Last of all you will need the tools of defense. These include guns, ammo, reloading components, explosives, warning devices, fireproofing, and traps, snares, and obstacles.

Please remember, however, that in my experience which now spans five continents and many, many years, *the best defense is obscurity, unobtrusiveness, and silence.* Rather than planning to shoot it out, plan to create the impression that your retreat contains no one and nothing of value. In the final analysis, this is the best way to protect what you must have to stay alive.

5. Getting to Your Retreat

CRISES SEEM TO FOLLOW ME around the world. My schedule once called for a thirty-day stay in India—starting the day the Chinese-Indian border dispute turned into a shooting war. Once, three days after I checked out of a hotel at the west end of Allenby Road in Tel Aviv, PLO terrorists moved in and killed eleven people. Then there was the time I was in London, waiting in Heathrow Airport, when renegade Iranians occupied their embassy.

If you like examples closer to home, I was once in Washington, D.C., talking to an Indian agricultural attache the day John Hinkley tried to shoot the President. When I went to Cuba in the late 1950s, I knew little about the revolution that was going on. By the time I left, the fighting had escalated to the point where Batista's position looked very precarious. Even in the U.S. I am not safe. I was visiting Boise, Idaho, when a backwoods trapper shot two game wardens.

I am concerned that trouble follows me around, so much so that whenever I travel now, it is with an ongoing concern about how I will get to my retreat if the collapse catches me in Belgrade, on the Island of Mindanao in the Philippines, in Odemes, Turkey, or wherever.

41

Israeli commandos got their people out of Uganda. Italian police rescued General Dozier from the Red Brigades. The British SAS routed those Iranians out of their embassy. Even the Canadians managed to smuggle our consulate people out of Teheran. But our government has, for ten years now, been staffed on the intermediate level by bumbling, uncomprehending drones who worry more about sexist language, seniority, equal rights, working conditions, compliance with their job descriptions, and the size of their vested pensions than they do about doing the difficult, disagreeable, but necessary job of protecting Americans' rights. There's a good reason why the Saudis keep money and property in the U.S., the French hoard gold, and overseas Chinese and Indian traders keep up extended familiy ties; they all have plans to get out of wherever they are when it becomes necessary. These are the self-rescue elements of those plans. Americans, too, need to pay attention to this concept of readiness and self-preservation.

We have already discussed the importance of establishing a retreat located on your home ground. I hope you agree now that you should never, under any circumstances, become a refugee. It doesn't take a genius to figure out that the equipment you store in your retreat can very easily provide the edge necessary to survive, and that good solid defense plans and preparations plus lots of determination can overcome some pretty significant odds.

But the cutting edge to all of this is *getting to your retreat,* out of the country, or to wherever you have established a safe refuge when the dislocations become severe, and it is no longer possible to travel by conventional means.

KNOWING HOW TO GET THERE

Until perhaps eight years ago, I was concerned about

this problem but had made few practical preparations to do something about it. Then I met Bill Munckin, who worked for the government in Saigon, Lima, and central Europe. I spent a good deal of time talking to him. He obviously knew what was going on. He had escaped from some pretty hairy situations, including Saigon at the time of its collapse. More important, he taught me that when the time actually comes to get out, it is going to be up to me to do it. There isn't much the U.S. government can or will do to help any of us, no matter how well connected we think we are, according to Bill.

Bill operated on the "Rule of Threes." It was his belief that the wise survivor will put together three separate, distinct evacuation plans, any one of which does not depend on the others, and each of which will work by itself if necessary. Doing this requires both an innovative evaluation of the means at hand and of one's own skills and talents.

For instance, when I travel internationally I carry quite a lot of cash, including some gold in a hidden money belt. In most cases nowadays, I cannot bring along any kind of weapon, but I know the cash will buy one if I need it. I also know that I will be able to use that weapon no matter what or where it is. That's a good, common application of the Larry Dring philosophy that what's between your ears saves your ass—not a bunch of hardware.

Bill Munckin is an experienced pilot who could, if necessary, fly a Lear jet or even a 727. One of his plans was to "requisition" a large transcontinental airplane. I can't do that, but I could fly a smaller plane a shorter distance and locate myself to finish the journey by other transportation.

Most survivors won't have to worry about 10,000-mile international "escapes," but there are a couple of lessons here. The first is that it is going to be up to you to seize whatever opportunity you can; you may even have to train yourself to get out. Not everyone can learn to fly a plane, but most people can. How about operating a boat, a motorcycle, a subway train, a bus, or a truck? If that's how you could travel in your area, you had better take some time now to watch the motorman run the train you take to work or have your brother-in-law show you how to operate his truck.

Every day each of us has an opportunity to see these types of vehicles. I suggest that from now on you don't just sit there, but learn how to run the damn things. Put yourself on a training program that will take advantage of every single opportunity you have in the coming years. If nothing else, it will make you more employable now with a greater range of skills after the collapse.

KNOWING WHEN TO GO

Second, be sensitive to what is going on around you. Interpret the news, don't believe it. Television, for instance, is a media of misinformation and hysteria. You will have to perceive the meaning behind the obvious and make your plans accordingly. I, for example, had no hesitation about leaving for Turkey in 1979 when a military takeover was imminent: I knew the army would stabilize the situation, not make it worse. Believe me, I didn't figure that out by watching the evening news. In this country, if we start seeing bank failures coupled with a breakdown in the food distribution system, watch out. These signs of social dislocation may well foreshadow an economic collapse.

Be especially attentive to veiled Soviet threats. They so outnumber us militarily that these occurrences are bound to increase dramatically in the near future. The Soviets' normal pattern is to orchestrate some sort of "incident," preferably through a Third World surrogate, and then capitalize on that situation. Traditionally the Soviets have attacked with massive amounts of men and armaments. Their general philosophy is that if you want your pants to stay up, use a belt *and* suspenders. This was their practice in Finland in 1940, on the eastern front in WWII, and now in Afghanistan, and it is the way they work when supplying weapons to the Syrians, Angolans, Cubans, Nicaraguans, and their other allies. On the other hand, Soviet equipment does not work very well and their plans often go astray due to lack of imagination, personal initiative, and flexibility.

It is my belief that any attack on the U.S. will be massive overkill in some places and irregular and extremely light in others. Their missiles and bombs won't function correctly, and as a result, some victims won't have a chance while others will barely be touched. This should provide some encouragement to urban survivors. If you are not at ground zero and have made some preparations, it won't be all that bad. Some missiles, I am sure, won't even arrive at their intended targets. Communications will be totally disrupted; the other side probably won't know for sure which targets have survived.

Edward Teller, who has worked for forty-three years developing our nuclear arsenal, made a good point when he reported in the *Wall Street Journal* that there will be time for the U.S. to evacuate if we see the Soviets evacuate. Obviously he is talking about the massive head-for-the-hills evacuation plans we are toying with. On the other hand, the Soviets, with their national shelter plans, will tip their hand if they actually start to implement them. The trick will be to monitor the BBC, French radio, or whatever. Even our media may catch on and be of some use.

At any rate, this chapter is about getting to your retreat, not predicting the collapse. Probably the best
easily obtained source of information in that area is the
better investment newsletters such as Douglas Casey's
book *Crisis Investing* (see bibliography). Read the papers
and watch the television news and read between the
lines. It is your duty to stay informed in a positive,
open, realistic way. Alarmist "Chicken Littles" won't
make it as survivors, either.

KNOWING THE RIGHT ROADS

If the real danger in your area is nuclear attack,
don't plan to evacuate by plane. In fact, your best plan
may be not to evacuate at all, but to pick the best walking route to your retreat—but don't pick just one route.
Have two alternatives in mind that can both get you
there. Some routes may be closed. You may have to
drive home through traffic-clogged streets or rough
neighborhoods if the collapse occurs while you are at
work. Perhaps you can ram a truck or bus through these
areas and make it safely. Just be aware of where you
might be and how you will get to where you want to be.

Bicycles are a great means of transportation if you
only have to go a few kilometers and no one will be
shooting at you. Bikes can get around and through ob-
structions that will block motor vehicles, but they are
slow, exposed, tough in bad weather, and can't carry
much. Motorcycles are better. They are miserable,
tough vehicles to operate but can nevertheless take you
great distances on little gas at great speed, and carry a
fairly respectable load.

What about getting the kids home from school? In
Africa the Rhodesians had a bus route, a car pool, and
armored car evacuation plans devised ahead of time in
case there was trouble. In the Congo the Europeans used

a special train to get out. The train was attacked and there were some losses, but at least they didn't mill around like a bunch of animals when the crisis occurred. They already had their plan worked out.

If a bridge might be out, plan to get around, over, or through it. If the freeways might be closed, know what you are going to do about that. You may even want to transfer jobs or move to a more convenient place in the same area. Even at my age I could walk 200 kilometers in three days if I had to! Maybe you need to get out with the wife and kids and develop that useful skill.

I keep forty liters of gas and an extra spare tie in any vehicles that are taken more than fifty kilometers from my retreat. Some of my regular job-related duties are within sixty kilometers of a large Air Force base. Whenever I am in the area, I am also ready to leave on five minutes' notice.

I figure I will have about an hour and a half to get out of the city after a nuclear strike. After that, the highways will be full of hysterical people driving to they don't know where. You might want to design a getaway vehicle. Perhaps you should buy a four-wheel-drive van for your business and install a heavy bumper and winch on the rig. Don't overlook public transportation, either. You may have access to school buses, company cars or planes, taxis, and trucks.

Be aware of unconventional opportunities. The last time I was in San Francisco I realized that I could simply walk out of the city along the subway tracks. Median strips between highways, waterways, park belts, and so on could all be used as evacuation routes.

If at all possible, keep your route short. Establish your retreat where you can easily get to it and not have to travel clear across the city in an area barred by rivers, overpasses, or whatever. Of course, this sword cuts both ways. If it is tough for you to get to your retreat, it will also be easier to keep others out.

The important thing is to admit to yourself you are going to have to do something and then make three sets of plans to do it. In my experience, nine out of ten Americans are frozen into inactivity by fear when a crisis occurs. Survivors must be in the top 10 percent, not the bottom 90 percent.

If necessary, establish some supply caches that you can use in an emergency to get through to your retreat. You might bury a .22 rifle, a pair of boots, ammo, some silver coins, a compass, and a rain slicker in the flower bed by your company parking lot. If the emergency arises while you are at work, you can dig the stuff up and use it to get to your retreat.

Survivors have to, I believe, commit themselves to dying with their faces to the wind if that becomes necessary. They have to develop a three-alternative escape plan. When the time comes, they will pick the best escape route under the circumstances and get on with it. The question of whether or not a collapse will really occur was settled when you devised your plan and built your retreat. The only real question is when the event will occur, and that is rapidly getting easier to predict.

The important thing to remember is that whenever you believe the time is at hand, act quickly and decisively. That's how people in Beirut, Afghanistan, and Cambodia made it—when it was time to move, *they moved!*

6. Retreat Location

THE LAY OF THE LAND HAS A tremendous bearing on how much energy the survivor will have to expend in defending his retreat.

Obviously topography and geography have a lot to do with the actual defense of your retreat from marauding bands. They also have a lot to do with defense against cold, hunger, wind, high water, drought, thirst, pestilence, and even insect pests and plant and animal diseases. That's why cabins were built where they were and cities grew up at the confluence points of rivers as collection areas for agricultural goods and regional food distribution centers.

Topography has a bearing on whether the survivor can even get to his retreat. What, for instance, will you do if you plan to hole up with your brother's family in the suburbs but you have to pass through a large population center to get there? It might be incredible folly to try to make it when everybody else is also on the road, or radioactive fallout is blowing from the direction in which you want to travel.

When you set up your retreat, remember that what you do now can minimize confrontation later. Pick a spot you can get to quickly and easily on turf that you are familiar with.

Be aware of the avenues of approach people might be tempted to use to get to your place. If these approaches are difficult or obscure, they may be easily defensible. One example is a sod house miles out on the prairie where no one would think of going, have the energy to get to if they did, or be able to find even if they did head out in that direction. An unwanted visitor would also be visible from three miles off if he did try to approach such a retreat.

Try to locate your retreat so that natural or man-made barriers will funnel movement away from your area. Use your imagination. You may have to dynamite a bridge or close a freeway off-ramp leading toward your retreat. This relatively simple expedient may keep the fleeing masses out of your neighborhood and make life much simpler.

AVENUES OF APPROACH

At the other extreme from the sod house, my dad lived through World War I in the basement of a church behind a huge pile of rubble in a back alley. The place met the test of obscurity, access, surveillance, defense, and was correspondingly difficult to get into and out of. It was a good, practical use of natural topography, even though the retreat was in the heart of a large city.

In Africa I ran across a Mennonite missionary couple who lived in a rural community on the east shore of Lake Victoria. They used to wear out a lawn mower every couple of months trimming the grass for several hundred meters around their compound. When the home folks whose donations supported these people found out about this extravagance, they severely criticized the couple. However, things are not always as they seem.

I cut the grass around my retreat because for three

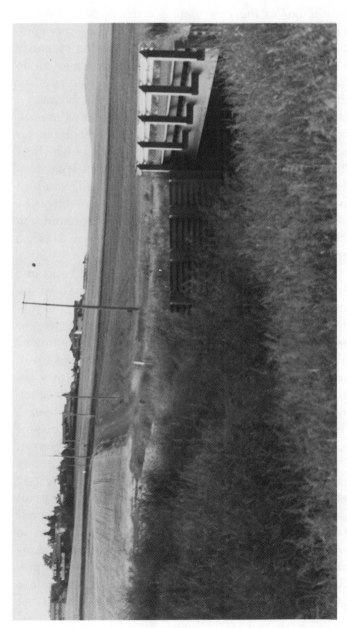

Blowing up a bridge leading to your retreat may not stop all foot-traffic in your direction, but it certainly will limit the number of vehicles that can reach you.

months out of the year there is a tremendous fire danger. Some not readily apparent but very real, very common danger may be your undoing if you don't identify it beforehand. Terrain and topography have a lot to do with what kind of surprises an enemy can deal you; they can also provide many surprises of your own making.

You may, for instance, build an extremely fire-resistant retreat but still roast in it when the buildings around you burn. Or what about collapsing high rises? They could bury you under tons of rubble. What happens if the gates on a dam are opened, leaving you high and dry? Will the broad prairie around your retreat be the scene of a tank battle, or will the high ground you occupy become an observation post or, even worse, a mortar position?

No retreat is absolutely unapproachable. I was in a bunker in southern Ethiopia that was attacked by Somali rebels. They crept up behind some rock and rubble under cover of darkness and started firing into our position. Coming in the previous day we had noticed this problem with the bunker and were prepared for it; we knew where the raiders would be when they attacked. As a response we fired into the rocks, ricocheting the rounds into their position; they soon retreated. This is an example of the small-scale complexities of using geography and topography to protect your retreat.

If possible, use the terrain to rig up some booby traps around your retreat. My book *Mantrapping* (see bibliography) covers that area pretty well, but one point I did not emphasize strongly enough is not to set your traps in such a way that they lead your adversaries to your retreat or convince them that there is something valuable in the vicinity that you are determined to protect. Again, obscurity and camouflage—blending into the local surroundings—is of immense importance. Traps

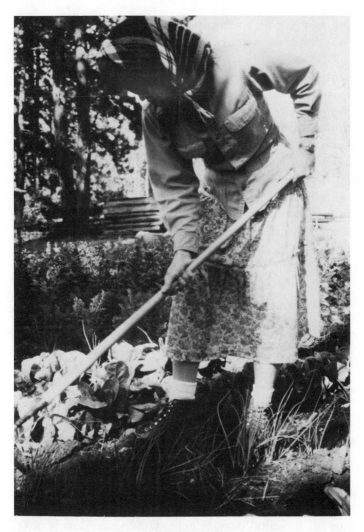

This woman is hoeing her survival garden. The garden, however, should be disguised by random planting. Straight rows are a sure sign of civilization.

and snares must conform to the land, not vice versa. You should remember to camouflage your garden as well. Don't plant in rows, weed with discretion, and plant root crops where the danger is high. In Africa we tracked down a lot of raiders by finding their gardens or livestock. Use the lay of the land to shelter your garden from suspicious eyes, not to advertise it. All of this assumes you have checked your area out and found a parkway, playground, backyard, or median strip with soil deep enough to grow a garden or raise some goats and rabbits. Virtually every survival guru, myself included, has had some kind of experience with survival groups who have their whole program worked out including the garden plot, except there is no life-supporting soil in the place these well-meaning folks have designated for their retreat. I usually recommend taking soil samples and analyzing them for nutrient levels before the land for a retreat is purchased.

USING THE TOPOGRAPHY

Natural barriers such as rivers, lakes, and mountains can provide a safe haven on one or two sides, or they can become the anvil against which you and your loved ones are battered to pieces. It all depends on how you secure your area and if, by some mischance, you get caught in the middle of some major action.

The natural topography can provide water, and it can be a source of fuel. City survivors may want to sweep off a section of street and catch the rain before it runs off downhill, for instance. Others may locate next to a pond or river, and use the barrier to both protect and provide.

Some survivors in Kentucky located their retreat on slate rock next to a stream. Behind them in the hill was a coal seam two meters thick running back God only knows how far. They occupied a renovated two-story brick store building on a little-used side street in the rundown section of a fairly large city. The water in the stream was polluted, but could be purified for use in a survival situation, and there was topsoil for a garden. The situation wasn't ideal, but no situation ever is. It was the people with their plan and initiative that made it workable.

Their big problem, in my estimation, was the high ground rising behind them on the hill. However, since there was no easy access up the hill, it is doubtful anyone would think to go up there unless the retreaters shot off their mouths.

One of the most effective harassment techniques I ever saw was in Cuba in the late fifties. Batista's forces had boxed in some of Fidel's followers in a rubbled, burnt-out area on the south edge of Matanzas. Even using planes, the government forces could not identify the rebels' central command area. The ground was too strewn with rubble for tanks or half-tracks, so the Fidelistas just kept sniping the army from irregular positions and held them off for weeks. The local people resupplied them whenever there was an especially dark night. Eventually the rebels were forced to leave, but it was a costly battle for Batista's troops.

In a survival situation, sniping can be an effective means of keeping intruders out, if it is carried out on a planned, intermittent basis over a large area. The idea is to create the impression that the area is unsafe and anyone who wanders into range may be fired upon. To do this effectively you must evaluate your area for these kind of possibilities and know how to move around the territory you control.

Many of the retreats that people plan, especially in the Midwest, are too damn cold. It *is* possible to live in northern Wisconsin, Michigan, or Minnesota, but it is not practical for city people who have never experienced 40 below in a log cabin before. Be aware of your limitations and the demands of the area where you will be living. City dwellers should stay in the city where fuel will be fairly abundant and live on stored food rather than freeze to death in the dark in one of our northern states.

Using the topography and geography of an area to protect yourself requires harmony with your surroundings. Work with them and not against them. Generally city people do best in the cities and country people do best in the country. That's why you should *never* become a refugee. Plan and equip your retreat in a place you know and then stay there till it's safe to come out and start rebuilding. Use the country; don't let it use you. That's the heart of the matter.

7. Who Is the Enemy?

BEFORE THE SURVIVOR CAN adequately defend his retreat, he must evaluate who, or perhaps even what, he is likely to have to defend it against. Without an accurate assessment of the dangers you may face, no matter how much work you put into your retreat, you may still find yourself ill-prepared to survive after the collapse. Two examples illustrate the extremes you might face.

What will you do, for instance, if the government sends Huey helicopters loaded with rockets and men to take your retreat? Can you withstand this kind of attack, and if so, how?

On the other hand, let us suppose there is a home for the retarded about a mile from your retreat. At the time of the collapse the workers, hearing you have shelter, come walking up with thirty wards in tow. Do you put a couple of bursts of M-16 fire into the group and send the survivors scurrying on their way?

If your answer is yes, how do you sleep at night or look yourself in the mirror afterwards? If your answer is no, then how do you accommodate the added number of dependent souls in your retreat? How do you feed them? What about sanitation? Obviously the enemy here is not necessarily the bloodthirsty mob so many survival gurus think it is.

During my tour in Africa I came across a village of about four hundred fifty Turkhana near Lake Rudolph that had been wiped out by Ugandan raiders. We found it from the air because of the many vultures flying around. Apparently the soldiers had surrounded the village and killed all of the adults with their rifles. Then they rounded up all the children and did them in by holding their faces in a fire. The old Africa hands said this was a commonly used technique, especially in the old days before colonization. We tracked the raiders for five days but never got close. They had a four-day head start and got fifty miles south into some heavily populated areas of Uganda before we could catch up with them.

Few people in the world would condone killing kids by stuffing their faces in a fire. On the other hand, the prepared survivor is likely to find himself in a similar moral dilemma unless he plans some countermeasures early on.

HAZARDS

The first and most dangerous enemies, in my opinion, are hunger and thirst. Then there are disease and freezing as a result of poor preparation against the cold. About ten years ago I went moose hunting up near Localsh, Ontario, with a fellow from Chicago who had never set foot inside a log cabin in his life. In the week we were together, he simply could not get used to the idea of getting up in the morning and building a fire in the stove to heat the room. All his life he had never had to do more than walk over and adjust the thermostat. After that experience I concluded that freezing

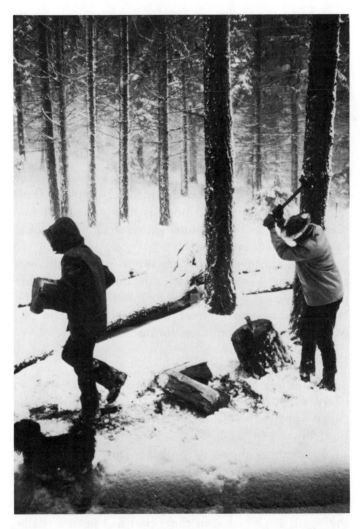

Being near a good source of fuel is an absolute must if your retreat is in cold country. Without wood or coal for heating and cooking, the danger of freezing is imminent.

may be the first and greatest enemy Americans will face.

The second group of hazards are NBC (nuclear, biological, chemical) agents. Since at least one of these risks is extremely likely to come up in a survival situation, the retreater will want to develop countermeasures against all three. These include an NBC-proof retreat, survey meters, dosimeters, decontamination suits, breathing apparatus, cleanup equipment, an appropriately shielded sleeping area, provisions for protecting food and water, and necessary medical supplies. That's the bad news. The good news is that you won't have many people poking around your retreat if any or all of these hazards are present.

Fire is another threat. City survivors especially need to plan either to avoid the fire, put it out, or just be fireproof. If you may run a risk of explosion, plan for that. Don't situate your retreat on the fourth floor of a wooden apartment building, for instance!

INTRUDERS

In terms of planning to deal with people who are likely to intrude, the first step is to discriminate between professionals (soldiers) and nonprofessionals (looters).

I remember the story (probably true) of the Frenchman who, after World War I, searched the globe for a place where he could live out his life in peace, quiet, and freedom. He settled finally on a remote island in the south Pacific that in times past had been a coaling station for tramp steamers. The man reasoned that with the advent of diesel-powered boats the place would fall into absolute obscurity, so he packed up his earthly goods and moved there.

The name of the island was Guadalcanal.

If you are likely to be in the path of advancing armies and can't relocate your retreat someplace else, your best plan is to button up and keep your head down. The Jews in the Warsaw ghetto found that out. Yet, to their credit, they held out weeks longer than anybody thought they could. Most military commanders know what happens when you back people to the wall in an absolute sense and avoid that situation!

In cities, mobs and their subsets—organized and random looters—will be the real problem for survivors. However, remember that these people must know you are there and believe you have something of value or your presence must constitute an affront to their collective ego. Mobs attack the presidential palace because of what it symbolizes, not so much because of any threat it might present or loot it might contain. Along with evaluating the potential for mob violence, you should also consider how well armed a potential mob might be. My rule of thumb is to assume they will be better armed than you might expect at first, but that they will use their arms poorly. Newspaper accounts notwithstanding, that's what is happening in Afghanistan and what happened in Lebanon, Budapest, and Tehran.

In the country, the human problem is generally squatters and refugees. Given current civil defense planning, it looks very much as though we will have tens of millions of people milling around in the country with no place to go. Rural survivors will face a far greater threat from these folks than city dwellers will from hard-core looters who deserve to be shot anyway.

Handling crowds of otherwise innocent people who have been hauled out to the country by the authorities simply requires that you keep them from even getting near your retreat. If they aren't around, you won't have

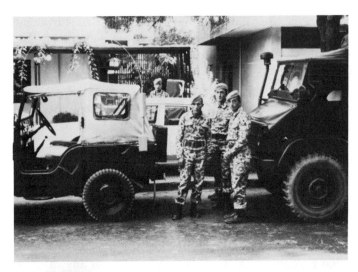

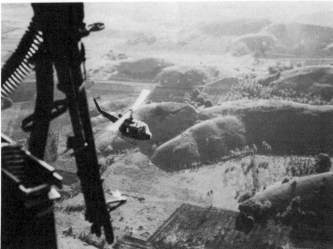

Factions of specially trained units like these elite Turkish Special Police (top) have the equipment to make retreaters' lives miserable. The helicopters (below) are looking for insurgents in the Philippines. The "enemies" retreatists face may be central authorities who want to quiet those people they perceive as a threat.

to make tough decisions about how to handle them. These people can generally be characterized as (1) stupid—they made no preparations for the collapse; (2) gullible—they believed governments could or would care for them; and (3) nonvigilant and nonthreatening truly desperate people who can only beg. They don't have the energy to riot.

There are some countermeasures you can take against the invading hordes, but pulling this off requires making preparations before the collapse occurs. What you're going to do is set out good booby traps and build defensive structures in which to place machine guns. Many good books on building booby traps exist. For perhaps the first eight years of the Vietnam war, we perceived these devices to be our greatest threat. The problem for the survivor is that all the plans require some kind of explosives. (They need not be military explosives, but they are explosives nevertheless.) Simple home production of booby traps is not hard for the reasonably clever survivor. Using homemade explosives, however, can make the task too dangerous to consider. Your best bet is to spend some time now learning how to use explosives and then store an adequate supply in your retreat for use when the time comes.

Burglars and thieves will be a problem for both urban and rural survivors. They can be handled initially with a warning system such as dogs, geese, or guinea hens, or an electronic alarm system until things stabilize enough to form protective associations. Sneak thieves are not brave people and will not relish the prospect of getting shot.

If your area is not physically damaged when much of the rest of the nation is, you will have a tough time with the local government who may want to confiscate your guns and send them to the front and distribute your food and supplies to the needy. Martial law is an insidious concept that allows government agents to confiscate all of your property and use it for their own purposes. I suspect that these are the same people who are currently running the antigun movement. Because they know that if we are allowed to keep our guns, they won't be able to run things, they know that they must disarm us before we need to use them. I have seen this happen in Africa, Asia, Central America, and Canada. I may have to die in the streets, but I will never die in somebody's jail because I lacked the means to protect myself.

One question I am frequently asked is what, or who, in the final analysis, is the most dangerous enemy? My answer is that if you know his capacities and equipment, and plan accordingly, no enemy is especially dangerous. The real danger comes from being surprised or unprepared for what might happen. Plan to control events; don't let them control you.

8. The Psychology of Defense

WITHIN THE SURVIVAL MOVE-
ment are a great number of gun buffs who seem to think
that it would be great fun just to jump from one firefight to the next. Invariably these are also people who
have never been in a shooting situation before, but that
isn't the issue I am concerned with at this point.

Let us suppose that you are safe in your retreat and
everything is working well. All of the jobs have been
assigned and things are going pretty much as you had
planned. The banks have failed, the farmers have not
gotten their crops in, much of our country's productive
capacity has been destroyed by government bungling,
and you are sitting there awaiting the time to come out
and start rebuilding. Let us further suppose that your
area is relatively free of people and no one really knows
you are there. Your patrols go out at regular intervals,
and in general you are in control of your lives, your
turf, and most important, your future.

Then, like a bolt from the blue, your road guard
calls in from a kilometer or so out to report that two
old women with perhaps ten small children are walking
up the road in the direction of your retreat. You think
about it for a moment but, unless your situation is
unique, you must conclude that it would be harmful in

65

the long run if the twelve newcomers became part of your survival unit.

Quickly you get back on the radio. You instruct your guard to remain hidden and allow the party of helpless, defenseless, and probably desperate waifs to pass by. Hopefully they will not discover your retreat or even tarry long in your area. But your hopes are in vain. After a couple of hours they spot your gardens and other signs of civilization and head straight for your retreat entrance.

What, pray tell, do you do now? Shoot them all? Take them in and jeopardize the health, safety, and viability of your unit? Refuse to acknowledge their presence while they plunder the garden? Turn the dogs on them? If they are average American kids (which is likely), they will have been raised on a diet of television. They can't work, have no discipline and, to make matters worse, appear sickly and are likely carrying at least one disease.

Any survivor who has not rehearsed this sort of scenario in his own mind has not really come to grips with the hard issues of defending his retreat. The one incident in Africa that I did not handle well and that stands out foremost in my mind was like this one. Situations like this are bound to come up time after time after the collapse. Country people will be inundated with refugees from the cities; city people will confront scores of helpless people wandering around trying to figure out what to do to stay alive. These folks are not going to be an active, immediate threat. Most won't even be armed. Take my word for it, doing them bodily harm is going to be incredibly, almost impossibly, difficult. How, then, are you going to handle the situation?

In Africa the tribesmen I was with handled the matter in the only way they knew; later even I became so hardened that what they did didn't bother me. But in this country with my own people, the problem is one whose solution still eludes me.

About all I can suggest is that you conceal your retreat well and try to keep these people away. When it's time to take out a bridge, close a road, cut down some trees, knock over a building, or whatever, don't hesitate—get out there and do the job. Procrastination and indecision have no part in a survivor's life-style.

A related problem is the potential conduct of your own unit in an actual fight. The U.S. military has determined that 75 to 80 percent of even well-trained front-line troops do not fire directly at the enemy. Pilots will shoot rockets at planes, mortar men will bombard a target area, but it's the rare individual who will, for instance, snipe directly at another human being. In Vietnam there was a constant need for American snipers armed with long-range rifles, silencers, and fiber optics sights to kill enemy soldiers. I met one fellow at the advanced marksmanship unit at Fort Benning who was reported to have made almost a thousand confirmed kills in less than three months. This would have been a cheap, easy way to fight the war except for one thing: the Army was unable to find more than a handful of people who had both the skills and the desire to personally do in that many of their fellow human beings.

In a survival situation, the circumstances will be far more precarious, but I would guess that no more than one in ten of the people with you will be able to shoot at an enemy with lethal intent. The others will waste their ammo firing into the air around the target at best; many will not be able to shoot at all.

An incident that occured during the Nez Percé Indian War in Idaho illustrates this point and also makes another. At the Battle of the Clearwater, General

Howard's cavalry surprised about six hundred of Chief Joseph's braves camped along the South Fork of the Clearwater River about ten kilometers south of the present-day town of Kooskia. Nearly five hundred soldiers dismounted and charged downhill from an eight-hundred-meter elevation toward the Indian camp three hundred meters below. They were supported by Gatling guns and pack howitzers.

The account is not completely clear, but certainly no more than fifty and perhaps as few as twenty-four Indian warriors counterattacked *uphill*, stalling Howard's advance. Thirty-five troopers were killed or wounded while the Indians lost four braves.

The point is that the Indians, numbering about six hundred, had already selected those warriors who would shoot troopers as opposed to those who would either only shoot *at* troopers or not at all. These picked men stalled the advance while everybody else stayed behind and packed camp.

People who do not shoot, or who shoot ineffectually, are not cowards. It's just that in almost every culture, the average person has an enormous emotional hurdle to clear before he will actually shoot someone. Certainly it is not immoral to shoot someone who is trying to take your life or deprive you of your supplies and the safety of your retreat. Someone has to fight, and hopefully someone will. You probably won't know for sure who that someone will be, but without this hope you yourself may perish.

It takes training, equipment, and a knowledge of the terrain to pull off something the way the Nez Percé did; but it must and can be done. Training sessions are the key, and they are also an excellent opportunity for you to learn who will do the job and who won't. You might be able to nudge the fence sitters in the right direction.

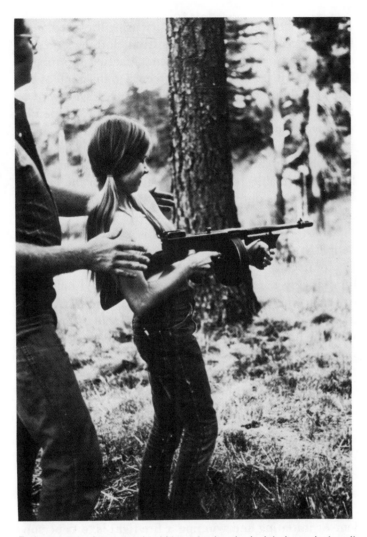

Each person in the retreat should be trained to do the jobs he or she is well suited for. Some people are not psychologically able to handle a gun. The girl pictured seems to enjoy learning to use this Thompson submachine gun.

I recommend weapons practice using life-sized, man-shaped targets; old mannequins from clothing stores are even better if you can get them. Practice shooting at these until it is second nature to engage this kind of target. The shooters will gradually become desensitized to the point where practice and reality blur. Hopefully they will become part of the actual fire team when the time comes. In the training process you will also find out who are the better marksmen, and who are most likely to be able to inflict casualties upon the enemy. Don't berate your people. Accept the skills they have and make do.

Another way of handling this problem is to ask people you think are potential warriors to shoot animals for food. Surprisingly few people actually kill anything hunting any more, and even fewer have lived on a farm or ranch where slaughtering for meat is common. Shooting a goat or two or some rabbits or chickens can be extremely helpful. This practice, if carried out with the right people, will tend to desensitize them to the act of taking life. Obviously it cannot and should not be done with members of your team who are irreconcilably repulsed by the whole process.

A point to remember is that in a real combat situation, it doesn't take many of the right people to handle the shooting. Also, don't forget that many (but not all) of those who might attack you are similarly prejudiced against killing.

Another very good method of dealing with the problem of initiating and winning a fire fight is to depersonalize the confrontation a bit. The best way to do that is to employ booby traps mixed with some good old battlefield psychology. Kurt Saxon's now dated book *Poor Man's Armorer,* as well as William Powell's *Anarchist Cookbook,* Bert Levy's *Guerrilla Warfare,* and the

Rhodesian Leader's Guide are all invaluable sources of information (see bibliography).

One method is to set trip wires hooked to mouse-traps that will trigger dynamite charges. If you know how, set out homemade or even store-bought mines to guard the open, easy approaches to your retreat. The idea, of course, is to get your adversaries to stumble into your traps and blow themselves up. (Just be sure your own people all know the safe approaches.) Another procedure is to set up manually operated antipersonnel devices similar to claymore mines, rockets, and electrically detonated charges.

A variation is to set up a remote-controlled perimeter system that allows you to detonate large quantities of easily made napalm behind your adversary after he has approached to a predetermined distance from your retreat. Most people, finding themselves cut off from behind, will beat a hasty retreat back through your mine field where other devices will hurry them on their way. Remember the attack-from-behind concept; it is exceedingly unnerving and does not involve the psychological problems shooting at people does.

One problem with these elaborate systems is they must be reset after each use and are subject to malfunction due to weather and age. Another problem will be policing the area after a battle; very few Americans are used to this kind of duty. In fact, many American survivors have never seen a corpse under any circumstances.

In the case of undesirable visitors whom you do not want to shoot at, presenting an unhealthy, unkempt appearance can be a deterrent. Have them confronted by a seemingly wounded, tattered member of your party who rants and raves crazily. Put out signs of death and destruction. Cover the area with smoke. Warn people of plague in the area. These are all worth a try, especially with old-women-and-children type intruders.

In a firefight, it is often helpful to give the impression that you have more firepower than you really possess. An old military axiom dictates that one should destroy the most dangerous threat at the greatest distance. Sometimes this is not possible. In Hungary in 1956, the freedom fighters displayed replicas of antitank weapons and kept the Soviets completely out of some sections of Budapest. You may, like the Hungarians, convince aggressors that the game is not worth the candle and keep their big hardware out of your area. When there is no other way, it's worth a try.

Every retreater who might face a paramilitary threat should have several semiautomatic weapons that can simulate machine guns. This requires ready-made, full-auto conversion devices and a number of spare magazines. The noise alone will probably discourage all but the most hard-core.

If at all possible, shoot to wound, not to kill. People approaching your retreat who suffer casualties will usually pull back carrying the wounded with them. After a bit they may lose interest in you and seek shelter elsewhere. If their resolve is stiffened, you still have an advantage: dead people can be left in a pile. Wounded require someone to stay and nurse them. Even the African Shifta took care of their wounded.

Untrained people who are fired on will panic and think of little else but getting out of danger, especially if there is some blood. This will also be true of your own group, so be ready.

In all of these situations, the thing to remember is that once authority is reestablished, you may be brought to trial for murder. There are varying degrees of seriousness in every situation. As a retreat leader you will have to evaluate each one using good common sense to make an accurate assessment. Don't kill people unless you have no alternative. Eventually some sort of law and order will be established, and you will almost certainly be held accountable for acts of extreme indiscretion.

What do you do, for instance, in a small town if the chief of police, whom you know well, sends a message to your retreat saying that he is sending along three families for you to put up? Readers who live in small towns know that this is a very real possibility. City people should understand that their country cousins have no easy answers when it comes to survival, only a different set of problems.

Executing and installing a predetermined, well-thought-through plan of defense for your retreat will provide a great deal of psychological comfort for your survival unit. They will resist attack with the confidence and determination that will get the job done.

Your task is to evaluate the equipment, training, and implementation requirements and get going *now* to assemble what you need. Don't forget that many of these needs are psychological, and that you, as the leader, will have to meet them. And don't forget, too, that if you don't start now, your cause is probably lost.

9. The Retreater's Arsenal

I LIKE LARRY DRING'S ARMA-
ments philosophy. For those who don't immediately
recognize the name, Dring is a soldier's soldier, a survivalist who has made it in Beirut against Soviet tanks, in
southeast Asia against "yellow rain," and in a dozen
other nasty little places that I can't mention in this
book.

I was at a conference where Dring was one of the
featured speakers. During one of the seminars a well-
meaning attendee asked Dring what guns he should take
to Honduras, where he was headed to do a bit of free-
lance combat. Dring's answer was so true and so to the
point that I wrote it down.

"It isn't the guns you take in your duffle bag,"
he said. "It's what you take between your ears that
counts. They have tons of guns, ammunition, and explosives; the bush is full of edibles. You don't have to take
a goddamn thing except training, preparation, and
knowledge.

Because the above is so true, I am going to break
with the blood-guts-and-guns crowd and tell you that
the first piece of equipment you will need is information about equipment. You may very well need guns,
explosives, booby traps, antihelicopter wires, and many

other things to protect your retreat. But you also must know how to use the core items you have laid back or cached. You will also absolutely have to know how to use captured or scrounged equipment. Heavy machine guns and antitank weapons, for instance, aren't ordinarily available to survivors, but when trouble comes, it will bring these weapons along. Then it will be imperative that you know how to get them and use them.

BOOKS

Because information is so vital, I have cataloged the major areas and recommended a few core reference books in each one. In all cases I have tried to keep the list as short as possible. However, we are still talking several hundred dollars, a sum that is going to be fairly tough for most readers. To ease myself over this hurdle a few years back, I made a list of all the books I had and then a list of all the books I felt I needed. My intention was to prioritize my purchases, which supposedly would then be made in an orderly fashion.

What actually happened was that I discovered some glaring holes in my library, especially in the medical information area. This was so unsettling that I immediately set out a couple of extra fox traps to raise the additional money to pay for the books I desperately needed. The general categories along with basic recommendations will be found in the bibliography.

WEAPONS

The second most important item in the retreater's arsenal is guns and ammo—not just any guns and any ammo, but a specifically tailored inventory of weapons that will do the job correctly when the time comes. You are going to be mighty foolish if, for instance, you buy several shotguns and your retreat is located on the flat,

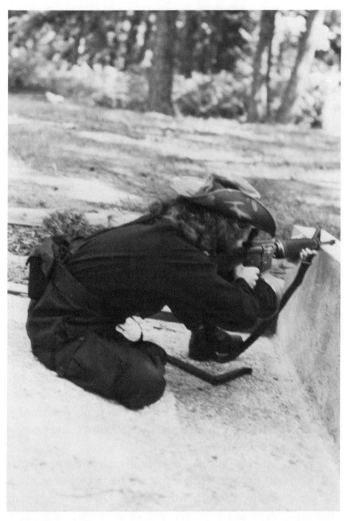

This retreatist is planning in advance what she will do with her M16 if she must resort to fighting in defense of her retreat. If you are going to stockpile guns and ammo, you had better devise an adequate strategy for using them.

open prairies of Illinois. If it is likely that you will face military or police personnel, you had better acquire something that you can convert to full-auto fire. City retreat defenders may want to consider purchasing something that will penetrate light armor—I have a .338 magnum with metal core solid bullets.

My first specific recommendation is that you acquire an accurate .22 rimfire rifle. One of the many good, solid bolt actions would be fine or, if you can find it, a good single shot. A .22 is easy to learn to shoot, quiet, inexpensive, durable, and in skilled hands it can be a lethal weapon against intruders. Another oft-cited advantage of a .22 is that it won't tear your wallet off your ass to lay back a couple of thousand rounds of ammo.

The next recommendation may surprise you, but a real necessity for defending your retreat is something to make explosives go off with—fuze, caps, primers, etc. Setting many booby traps, taking out bridges, roads, buildings, etc., all require detonators. Through all of my years kicking around the world, I have had little trouble improvising explosives using fertilizer, petroleum products, industrial chemicals, and even household cleaners. The primers and fuzes were always the problem, though, especially because homemade detonators are notoriously unpredictable.

Fuze can be purchased virtually anywhere. Electric and conventional blasting caps are hard to get in cities, but reasonably easy in rural areas. Do some planning now to decide how many you will need, then get to work acquiring that amount for your cache. We are talking about twenty or so dollars and some time and effort, surely a small price to pay.

My next priority is a military rifle for every member of the retreat group who will be actually engaging any attacker. Don't kid yourself about this one. If your wife isn't going to defend against intruders, don't waste money buying a gun for her—buy another case of ammo for the guns you will be using.

Good military rifles are horribly expensive, but because they are rugged and reliable and parts will be easier to find, I suggest you bite the bullet. Get something like an FN assault rifle, an AR-15, or H&K 91 or 93. Be sure to buy a rifle that fires readily available military ammo. In this country, for instance, I am leery of the new Egyptian AK-47s, because the 7.62 x 39 mm rounds they fire are hard to get in the U.S.

If you already have a good hunting rifle in a military caliber, you might skip this acquisition until your other needs are met. However, many commercial hunting rifles are odd calibers and are subject to breakage and malfunction in paramilitary use. I saw five men die at the hands of Somali Shifta in the town of South Horr in northern Kenya, in part because they relied on hunting rifles. The popular lever action rifle that so many people own is a poor choice for survival use. In a firefight, lever action users will be at a distinct disadvantage, even if their guns don't break down after a couple of dozen rounds. Commercial rifles can be used for sniping, but so can properly equipped military rifles. In addition, don't forget that many hunting guns are extremely inaccurate.

In any case, you should lay in a good supply of ammo for your guns; I suggest laying back 1,000 rounds. For commercial guns of unusual caliber, it might be wise to put back twice that much, depending on that particular gun's intended role. You can hold down the cost of stocking ammo by buying surplus rounds or by reloading components. Another suggestion is to keep your eye peeled for surplus brass, bullets, and primers. If you use good common sense and are willing to look around, you can save some additional bucks here.

Be warned, however: you will need whole ammo to defend your retreat when the howling mob turns up your street, not bullets, primers, and powder sitting on the workbench. That's not the time to start screwing the dies into the press while your wife gets out the powder scale.

I'm a fair pistol shot, so my next item is a good handgun. Buy one for every third or fourth member of your defense group. More pistols than this may be fun, but they're not really necessary or practical; there just aren't that many people who can shoot them well. If you don't set limits you will end up expending all your ammo firing pistols to little effect.

Which pistol to get is a good question. Those who can shoot a pistol well get along very nicely with a .22 rimfire. On the other hand, I can consistently hit a half-meter target out to 150 meters with my 9 mm because I have practiced so much with my .22. It's the chicken-and-egg syndrome. I can't tell you which pistol to get first, a .22 or a center fire. Should you get a big gun to signal with and use in emergencies at close range or a .22 to practice with? The only point I would make is that virtually every really good pistol shot learned with a .22.

At any rate, if you do buy a pistol or pistols, get modern, well-made automatics. No one uses revolvers for military purposes now. Other than .22s, you won't even be able to get ammo for revolvers. Do get a fully enclosed flap holster and at least two extra magazines, and store your extra ammo in the magazines, not loose in your pocket.

Two items I don't have much use for are shotguns and submachine guns. Shotguns have no range or penetration and are easily defeated. Some survivalists think they will hunt with their shotguns after the collapse; in fact they will either starve to death or die at the hands of a guy with a .22 who steps back and snipes at the shotgun user. Hunters consume more calories than they collect; hunting *is not* a valid survival technique. You can test the validity of my theory regarding shotguns by asking yourself what is the one weapon a dictator will allow his citizens to own. It is a shotgun because shotguns as military weapons are virtually worthless.

Submachine guns are inaccurate ammo burners. The trend worldwide is toward shortened assault rifles such as the CAR-15 or the Valmet Bullpup rather than submachine guns. These .223 caliber weapons are really deadly; they are also fairly accurate, light in weight, and basically trouble free. At long range, however, they leave much to be desired.

EXPLOSIVES

Next, take a look at your explosives situation. If you can't obtain commercial or military explosives, lay back the appropriate chemicals. I keep three or four cases of dynamite around; lacking that, I would lay in some forty kilo bags of ammonium nitrate, some diesel fuel, and so on. You will also need chemicals like potassium permanganate, glycerine, steel wool scouring pads, chemicals with which to make acetylene gas, bottles of LP gas, gasoline, or whatever else you intend to use for barriers and booby traps.

Don't forget trip wires, posts, shovels, disposable containers, batteries, road spike setups, and all of the other gear and paraphernalia it will take to put your stuff in. This hardware will include front-line material such as wire barriers to keep out helicopters.

Other items people usually forget when planning

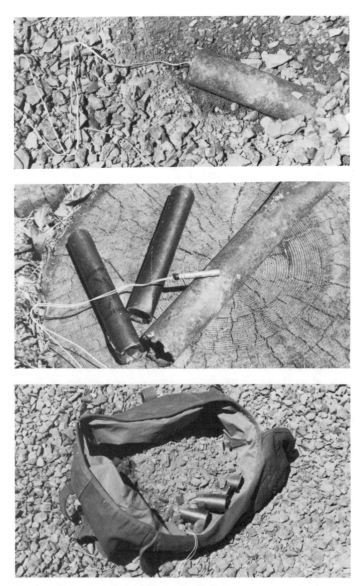

An electrically fired stick of dynamite planted in a road bed (top) can be an effective deterrent. Electrically fired dynamite can be rigged in pipe to make nifty pipe bomb (center). Dynamite buried in a rock-filled satchel and hung in a tree makes a devastating explosion.

their retreat defense are bulletproof vests and two-way radios. Modern, lightweight flak jackets are readily available at moderate cost. If you have the money, pick up one or two.

Radios and communications gear in general are essential. I have switched from handheld CBs to two-meter walkie-talkies made in Japan. I also have a set of battery-operated intercoms to use in my retreat. If you can't talk to your people, you won't be able to direct your retreat defense; keep that in mind.

The last items are military hardware such as anti-tank mines, hand grenades, rocket launchers, claymore mines, heavy machine guns, and the like. There is a lot of this stuff around, but currently it is kept out of sight. After the collapse, it will reappear. Be aware of what there is and how to use it. Also make an inventory of what items you feel you will need given what may be used against you. Buy the technical manuals for the stuff now. When the need arises, it will be easier to get what you need if you know what you want and how to use it.

Recently while on assignment on the Island of Mindanao in the Philippines, I ran across a group of Moros who had a couple of interesting improvised weapons. In one case they took standard rifle-launched parachute flares, opened the end, took out the star shell, and packed the cavity with dynamite. The Moros had become very proficient at lobbing these grenades into the windows of buildings, under Jeeps and into foxholes. Used this way, they were highly effective.

Another interesting weapon was a mortar made from 3 1/2-inch water pipe capped on one end and with two swinging legs attached to a collar. They fired the thing with a sawed-off 12 gauge shotgun brazed to the tube's bottom. For rounds, they used no. 6 vegetable cans half full of dynamite covered with cement. The fuze was standard dynamite fuse with a regular cap. About one round in five didn't go off. The Moros claimed they had never had a premature detonation.

Another weapon to seriously consider if you can afford it is a light machine gun. Semiautos that have been custom-altered melt down with terrifying ease. Unless you really know what you are doing, I cannot recommend one.

Weapons standardization is extremely important and implicit in everything in this chapter. Several years ago I took the step of standardizing my hunting guns. This minimizes ammunition and maintenance problems and reloading is simpler. Keep standardization in mind for all your guns, not just the rifles.

Having said all of this, let's recall my original premise: blood, guts, and guns are not going to protect your retreat. Your own skill and intelligence are the things that will do that. You won't miss anything by staying out of a firefight.

10. Beyond Firepower

THE SUBJECT THIS CHAPTER EX-
plores is one we have nibbled around on several times
previously without coming to any conclusion. It centers
around my firm belief that the survivor should follow
the old Roman military philosophy and plan for war; by
so doing, he is most likely to enjoy peace. Fight if you
must, but try your utmost to orchestrate events so that
confrontation is absolutely the remedy of last resort.
Then if you do get into a fight, unload with everything
you have. Don't handle this last responsibility half
heartedly.

My approach to this issue is not particularly ortho-
dox, yet it has served me well for a number of years: it
is to ask the question, "How far can my enemies walk?"
I am referring to the two-legged kind of enemy and not
to the broad spectrum of hunger, cold, and disease that
might undo the survivor.

Military personnel can generally walk farther than
any other group. Mechanization notwithstanding,
soldiers still wear out a lot of shoe leather. For this reason, trained, organized soldiers constitute a threat to the
average retreater. Still, if they want to occupy your retreat, they will have to do so on the ground, even

though they may have effective means of harassing you and making you keep your head down from afar.

On the plus side, the military must as a general rule have a good reason for wanting to occupy your retreat, and their reason will usually have to be of a higher order than that of a looter or common thief. The military would not, for instance, be particularly interested in seizing the year's supply of food you have stored at your retreat, even if they were sure beyond a reasonable doubt that the supplies were there. Food for, say, five people is not much to hundreds of soldiers who generally have their own rations anyway.

On the other end of the spectrum, most people, especially Americans, cannot and do not walk very far, especially if they have to carry food, water, weapons, and clothing along with them. Accounts of the San Francisco earthquake and the Chicago fire also documented the fact that people under stress do strange things. In these cases, as they evacuated their homes, people took with them bird cages, vases of flowers, bootjacks, and other worthless items. Not only could they not walk far, these folks further encumbered themselves with unimportant, impractical baggage.

A number of people have told me that they intend to keep the masses away from their retreats by dynamiting a key bridge or two. If they can do the job a mile or so from their retreat, they will have done a lot to secure their areas. People just aren't going to walk very far, especially if they don't know where they are going or why they are going there—another good reason to maintain secrecy about your retreat's location.

Creating obstacles and barriers to your retreat can take different forms; be alert to the possibilities and use whatever is at your disposal. It might be a body of water, burned-out buses and trucks, piles of rubble, downed electrical lines, a large truck or even a really gung-ho retreat group that will duke it out with intruders ahead of you and save you the effort. It is extremely important to disguise your comings and goings as much as possible. Don't, while hostilities are raging, enter or leave during the day. Don't allow raiders or other combatants to operate out of your retreat unless you are absolutely certain they won't be captured and that whatever confrontation they precipitate will happen well out of your own area. Sometimes it may seem necessary to violate this rule, but give it a second thought; there is always a way to handle the situation without sacrificing the integrity of your retreat.

Don't fire from your retreat unless absolutely necessary and then do so from hidden, scattered points within your area that are difficult to pinpoint. Most retreats will be buttoned-up affairs and not bunkers. Given the need to protect against NBC threats, there may be no place to shoot from unless an attacker actually comes in the front door. As I have previously said, pick a retreat location that will be obscure and inconspicuous and then use all your creativity to camouflage it so that it stays that way.

Use subterfuge if necessary. For instance, erect large official-looking signs warning all that approach that the area has dangerously high radiation levels. In cities similar signs or others announcing the presence of chemical warfare agents, plagues, diseases, or whatever would be effective.

If you can't use explosives, consider buying fifty pounds of roofing nails to spread on the roads, or stringing some heavy electrical wires around. I saw these used with incredibly good effect on Mindanao in the Philippines; even the helicopter pilots wouldn't go near the wire, for fear of being electrocuted or tangled up in it.

One of the most important don'ts regarding retreats is don't allow your place to become the nerve center for any kind of resistance movement unless it is a question of last resort. This is true even if there is no shooting. An enemy will always go after the headquarters if they can locate it. Nonprofessionals like ourselves will soon be located and become the targets of some highly professional military action.

Since the best retreat location is your own home, look for a remote, nondescript homesite location, either in the city or the country. You might consider moving to a less central, less traveled area if that's what it takes. This may be the most important thing you do as part of your future defense needs.

Moving to a better location is not an outlandish idea; the typical American moves, on the average, every 3.2 years. Right now there must be thousands of aware survivors who are moving as a matter of course. If you're one of them, make the retreat potential of your new homesite an important criterion when picking out a place to live. Look for masonry buildings with basements or locations that have ready access to basements.

The most dangerous people I have run into have been ex-military types who roamed the country after the collapse of authority. Without a central command to control them and possessing modern equipment and the skill to use it, they were definitely a force to be feared and avoided. I saw them in Somalia, Uganda, Rhodesia, Laos, Cambodia, and North Yemen among others. To these people your relatively small cache of food, medicine, fuel, and weapons is a worthwhile prize. Thirty years ago I would never have believed that such people could exist in this country; today I don't know. Our government has created a vast welfare class who believe that being given food and shelter is their right. I suspect that many of these people are now in the military. Unchecked and uncontrolled, they could present a major threat.

The best defense against this type of person, both in the city and in the country, is thorough knowledge of the territory over which you will be operating. If you can get behind these people to harass them, you may discourage them enough so that they will leave. This is especially true if you learn to operate on your home turf with impunity at night. Under cover of darkness, a few people can move farther with greater impunity than they ever could in daylight. The North Vietnamese proved to be masters at this game. Before them, the Israelis developed entire battle plans based on decisive nighttime movement of small units. Yet, most people are basically fearful of the dark. They don't operate well in that environment.

Many years ago my Uncle Dugan told me about his experiences in the South Pacific during World War II. His outfit was made up mostly of farm boys from northern Indiana, Illinois, and southern Wisconsin. Quite a few of them were coon hunters and enjoyed swapping stories about tearing around the countryside from dusk till dawn trying to find their dogs.

It occurred to Uncle that these guys could be organized into a hell of a reconnaissance and patrol outfit. Most people are afraid of the dark; these guys loved it. They moved around as well at night as most people do during the day. They wound up spending hundreds of hours harassing the Japanese and enjoying every minute of it. When they encountered a superior force or one that tried to expose them with flares, they simply withdrew. Uncle said that the enemy fire often went on until dawn while his outfit was safe and sound in another sector.

The advent of sophisticated, mass-produced booby traps and good night-vision devices has now limited the advantage people like the coon hunters enjoyed. But I don't believe that the survivor need worry much about these unless he makes himself too much of a nuisance, and certainly not with renegade soldiers operating on their own.

Make sure the ancillary trappings of your retreat, such as domestic animals, gardens, and water collection facilities, are camouflaged. In Africa we often used these signs to determine how many people were in the area we were patrolling. Most Africans refused to abandon their cattle, even if it meant their lives. We simply tracked the cows to their hideout. Stock should be kept in camouflaged pens during the day and only turned out to graze at night and then only under close supervision. The pens should be located far from the retreat itself.

Don't stack up wood in a pile or hang wash out to dry. Keep trash and refuse hidden, not only to disguise your location, but to protect it from scavengers.

In some cases it won't be hard to protect your retreat. If the collapse occurs as a result of nuclear war and if the area is contaminated with radioactive fallout, chemicals, and biological agents, you can expect few visitors. On the other hand, you had best be prepared with decontamination suits, dosimeters, and Geiger counters to do at least some patrolling.

As I said at the beginning, your objective is to pick a spot out of the mainstream of activity and conceal your presence. Then, hopefully, you will not have to shoot it out with intruders. No matter how skilled and how well armed you are, the more often you have to shoot, the greater risk you run of getting shot. There will always be someone out there who is bigger and tougher than you are. Your job is to avoid meeting them.

11. Making It Difficult

ONCE YOU HAVE PICKED YOUR retreat site, improved and hardened it based on your assessment of the danger you may face in the future, and stocked it with the necessary items to stay alive for a couple of years, your next step is to do some things now to make it more difficult to break your retreat later. Here I am talking about the moat-and-drawbridge approach rather than screening and camouflage. This sort of defense must be planned and constructed ahead of time. It will be too late to dig the moat when the Huns are already climbing the wall.

One of the most effective means of offsetting the technological advantage that determined, practiced, plundering bands have in a survival situation is smoke. Many years ago when I was in Cuba, I frequently saw Castro's guerrillas effectively use smoke to prevent Batista's air force from hitting their positions. The guerrillas made large fires and piled them high with palm fronds and tires. The smoke shrouded the dank underbrush so much that it was virtually impossible for the pilots to pinpoint their targets.

In Vietnam the Viet Cong and North Vietnamese pulled the same trick. Smoke was the simple expedient with which they foiled our $25,000 smart bombs. With zero ground visibility, optically sighted, laser-guided bombs were worthless.

The Sulu Sea pirates used smoke to foil the Philippine coast guard. They rigged a heavy steel plate in the back of one of their boats with a propane stove underneath. By spraying light fuel oil on the hot plate, they were able to generate a huge smoke screen on just a little boat. The ploy was abundantly successful; they fired up the smoke generators going into and around small island bayous and channels, making it impossible for the good guys to follow. Survivors could do the same thing using a hot car muffler or exhaust manifold and a supply of oil.

However, smoke only works for a while, and it can also reveal the location of your retreat, especially if it is used too early in an engagement. Smoke is best used in conjunction with natural obstacles. That way, you deny the enemy the ability to shoot you or blow you up from great distances. When attackers are forced to slug it out at arm's length on territory familiar only to you, the game loses much of its glamor for them.

Natural obstacles can be a number of things. When I was younger, I remember two blocks of gas main blew up in Chicago, creating a huge impediment for man and vehicle. The same thing could be done intentionally to create a traffic-free zone in a large city.

Hills and valleys can be obstacles to attackers, especially if you can cover their approaches with something tough to get through like spiny blackberry bushes or thorny raspberries. Just remember that you also have to cover these military sand traps with adequate firepower.

The purpose of these obstacles is to slow an enemy on foot long enough so you can take some good shots at him. Tracked and tired vehicles won't be slowed a second by natural obstacles alone. Either rig heavy explosives in the approaches that can be traversed by vehicle, or better yet, use the natural terrain plus any other obstacles you can create to keep vehicles as far from your doorstep as possible.

Ideally the area around your retreat itself should be obscured by brush, landform, or rubble. The surrounding terrain must either afford you clear fields of fire or channel the enemy into them. Further back, the approaches should be taken out as a precaution against heavy equipment.

Water can also be a natural obstacle. At one point in our pursuit of some Congolese rebels, they diverted a small stream across the road and stopped our vehicles in the middle of a huge swamp—it was an extremely clever trick. Some retreaters in Tennessee plan to soak a clay hillside with water and drop the ground down onto the road. Their plan can and would work in a lot of places with steep hills, mountains, and water.

A great many traps can be made from rocks, logs, ropes, wooden trip levers, and other naturally occurring materials. The required tools can likewise be of the simplest type. The beauty of these traps is that they make ordinarily difficult terrain absolutely deadly to cross. In addition, the entire philosophy becomes organic. You become aware of the myriad possibilities of enhancing the natural obstacles around you, and by knowing how to trap an enemy, you are protected against falling into their snares yourself.

Urban retreaters can break out large chunks of concrete in the streets, pile cars on the approaches and even do little things like removing manhole covers so vehicles have to slow down and pick their way along.

The ideal situation is to cache explosives even if they are nothing more than industrial or agricultural grade dynamite. Then the survivor can build some genuine booby traps that will stop even a tank. My favorite one is made with a mousetrap, a battery, an electrical blasting cap, and a couple of sticks of dynamite. If you have time beforehand, put the dynamite in a tin can and fill it with cement. If not, use nails, glass, and bits of iron and stones in a bag with the dynamite.

A booby trap developed by the IRA can double as a hand grenade. They put half a stick of dynamite in a half liter tin can and fill it with cement. The fuze is made out of 8 cm of car antenna, a shotgun shell primer, a length of fuze, and a blasting cap; the spring detonator is made from parts of a rat trap. These devices have endless applications. They can be dropped from trees or buildings by remote control, rigged on trip wires, buried in roads, even floated down streams with a dissolving sugar cube to release the striker.

In the southern Sudan, we set up some bottles of gas on top of a couple of sticks of dynamite. Our initial plan was to set off the dynamite with rifles; later we got more sophisticated and rigged the charges with electric caps. One liter of gasoline has the explosive power of about eighteen sticks of dynamite if mixed properly with oxygen. Here again, we didn't get a chance to try our booby traps.

Explosives don't always have to be set up to kill. I believe I could keep random looters out of an alley leading to a city retreat by placing single stick charges shoulder high and detonating them with a trip wire. The blast would deafen the intruders and discourage further movement into the area.

One of the most feared devices is fire. Booby traps that use burning gasoline, oil, or even napalm, if you know how to make it, are extremely effective. We tried using fire to defend a farm retreat in northern Israel just after the Six Day War in 1967. Our plan was to

Booby Trap Defense Perimeter

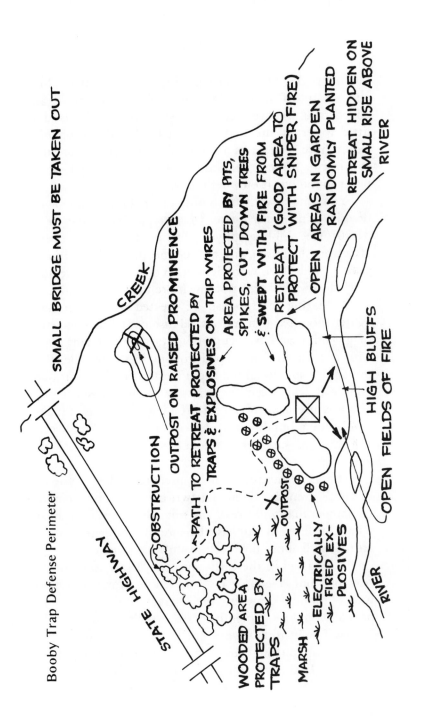

SMALL BRIDGE MUST BE TAKEN OUT

STATE HIGHWAY

CREEK

OBSTRUCTION

OUTPOST ON RAISED PROMINENCE

PATH TO RETREAT PROTECTED BY
TRAPS & EXPLOSIVES ON TRIP WIRES

AREA PROTECTED BY PITS,
SPIKES, CUT DOWN TREES
& SWEPT WITH FIRE FROM
RETREAT (GOOD AREA TO
PROTECT WITH SNIPER FIRE)

OPEN AREAS IN GARDEN
RANDOMLY PLANTED

RETREAT HIDDEN ON
SMALL RISE ABOVE
RIVER

WOODED AREA
PROTECTED BY
TRAPS

OUTPOST

MARSH

ELECTRICALLY
FIRED EX-
PLOSIVES

HIGH BLUFFS

OPEN FIELDS OF FIRE

RIVER

dump two 1,100 liter barrels of gas and oil down a hill and set it off with a flare pistol from a boat. As an added measure, we wet the hillside down and mixed a little water in the barrels of fuel. The plan probably would have worked as a last-ditch effort and as a signal for rescue forces. Thankfully, no one attacked, so I never found out if our method was sound.

You may want to consider making napalm as described in *Special Forces Operational Techniques* (FM 31-20) (see bibliography). This mixture is especially effective when used with a glycerine, potassium permanganate, and steel wool igniter. You can detonate the stuff electrically using nothing more than a light bulb.

A blazing inferno can be created using a butane lighter mounted beneath a steel dish containing one cup of glycerine and two cups of potassium permanganate with a plain steel wool pad floating in the middle. Rig the lighter so a weighted trip wire starts it. In about one minute it will warm the mixture enough to set it off. The mixture in turn can set off a jug of napalm or plain gas. Inside a building this device can be very disconcerting. Just be sure the ambient temperature is 65°F or less.

The same mixture can be used to make a type of thermite grenade. Keep the two chemicals in separate containers that will break and mix when thrown against a hard surface. In this case, be sure the ambient temperature is well above 65°F or the stuff won't go off.

In Pakistan in the early seventies, I saw some survivors put out a couple of dead horses; for about two weeks nobody came up their street. I thought these people would permanently destroy their sense of smell. Things finally didn't work out in this case, but for the right group putting out a dead pig or cow might be effective. In the city you might try throwing small rocks

Retreat Path Guard Snare

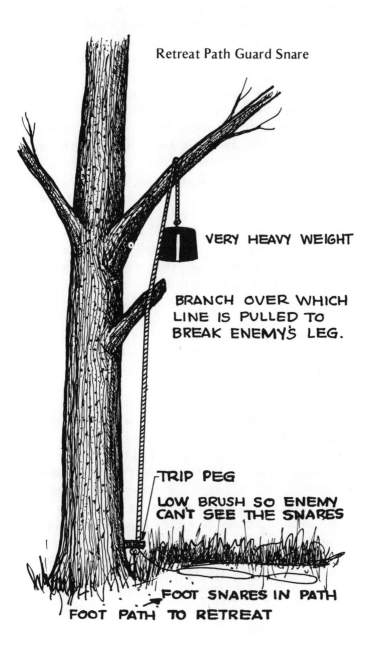

VERY HEAVY WEIGHT

BRANCH OVER WHICH
LINE IS PULLED TO
BREAK ENEMY'S LEG.

TRIP PEG

LOW BRUSH SO ENEMY
CAN'T SEE THE SNARES

FOOT SNARES IN PATH

FOOT PATH TO RETREAT

about the size of a goose egg off high buildings from irregular, unpredictable places. Keep them small in size. This ploy will greatly discourage anyone from entering your area unless they are pretty sure what they want to do.

Be wary of the approaches to your retreat. Make certain you have hidden revetments with a clear field of fire from which to fire to guard the area. If you think your area might be overrun, develop a plan for holding out inside your retreat itself. This may be nothing more than a way of selling your life to the highest bidder, but if you resolve to make them pay the price, it won't be long before the enemy runs out of bidders. If trained, disciplined military people get on top of your retreat, things are simply not going to go well. You may hold out for a while, but eventually they will overrun even the best, most well-designed retreat.

In the case of random mobs or looters, stopping them at the door will be a powerful deterrent. The problem is that some of your capacity to feed, heat, and protect yourself against NBC threats will probably be lost. Better, if possible, to keep them out of your area in the first place.

At the very least, lay out unobtrusive obstacles to force attackers to move up open approaches into your field of fire. Simple ploys like setting hundreds of sharpened two-meter long sticks into the ground at an angle can help enormously. Trees can be felled or glass scattered on the street. People hate to walk on crunchy glass even with shoes. In the Congo we broke tens of thousands of beer bottles along the approaches and in some ditches leading to our strong point. On the street, the glass crunched when the enemy approached. In the ditches it was just another little inconvenience that made keeping their heads down while we were shooting at them a bit more uncomfortable.

Something I want to try someday is putting grease on the pavement on a hilly street, on the stairs and sidewalk around my retreat, or anywhere else it might be nice to have someone slip and fall. Under the right circumstances this trick might have real merit; I just haven't found the right place yet.

There are a lot of things the retreater can do to improve his situation. The trick is to develop a knack for identifying them. Just remember, your job is to make life difficult for the intruder by using firepower, smoke, explosives, obstacles, snares, booby traps, and natural terrain.

12. What if It Comes to a Fight?

I MAKE NO APOLOGIES THAT the information in this chapter is simple and intended for basically nonmilitary persons who, having been pushed to the wall, find they have no alternative but to fight back. A survival group is, after all, not a military organization. It cannot really afford to take casualties. Those it does take will be family and close friends, perhaps even the retreaters' wives and children. Sustaining a survival group is not like commanding a company of soldiers or even patrolling with friends.

If the retreaters do suffer casualties, they will have violated the fundamental purpose of their group—to survive. These people have, after all, banded together to stay alive, not to outshoot someone in a firefight. On the other hand, another compelling reason survivors form retreat groups is to maintain their freedom. Many, many times individuals choose to sacrifice their lives rather than their freedom. I suspect that, apart from survivalists, most Americans have forgotten this.

In that regard, I especially appreciate the comments made by Aleksandr Solzhenitsyn who wrote *The Gulag Archipelago* (see bibliography), "Why didn't we fight? If we would have all individually resisted, many of us would have died, but we were doomed to die anyway, and it wouldn't have been so easy to send us to the camps."

A war of attrition works both ways. Tyrants very easily find that they are unwilling to pay the price of their power. Someday you may remember this when, with your supplies running low and the enemy coming over the inner wall, someone asks, "Do we surrender or do we take as many of them with us as we can?"

I have seen the same situation the world over which is why I urge you not to ever fall into somebody else's hands. Don't ever become a refugee! Without the means to defend yourself, you will die a thousand times rather than just once, just as you would if you resolved to duke it out with your attackers.

The plan I recommend for defending a survival retreat is one we worked out in Africa. Although it does, of course, have some elements of common military thinking, we used it quite a few times with untrained, thoroughly demoralized, unskilled people, usually with good results. The only real exception was among the Somali who were so warlike that the only thing they knew was to attack. Generally the plan works as follows:

1. Identify the group that will be part of the retreat defense.

How many young men, older men, able-bodied women, and trainable children can you count on? Before you go off half-cocked and start making assignments, take a moment to step back and see what you actually have. Be realistic about this assessment; evaluate how your people will really react under pressure.

2. Identify skills and talents.

I call this the "Chamber of Commerce" mentality. Whatever you have to work with, be it very good or awfully poor, it is what you have to work with. There is no sense bewailing the fact that you don't have a medic, a first-class sniper, or a gunsmith. Plan in an uncompromising, uncomplaining way to work with what you have. The idea is to get the job done using whatever talent is available. Perhaps the mix is unconventional or the strategy less than perfect, but get on with it. Don't sit around wishing things were different.

Doing all this requires that you start early on finding out what your people can and cannot do. Which kids can load magazines? Who is not sickened by the sight of blood and can therefore take care of the casualties? Who knows something about explosives, who can see the best in the dark, who can patrol, and so on?

3. Formulate a plan of action.

Know where the guns, ammunition, and explosives are, how they will be used, which approach route the enemy is likely to use, how they are likely to approach, and what your response will be when they do. Be aware that you will not react the same way to a tank, for instance, as you would toward some renegade soldiers or a howling mob.

4. Rehearse your plan.

Have many practice sessions and dry runs. Go through the various plans on a regular schedule till everyone acts by pure reflex and can do so very quickly. If possible, organize some actual shooting sessions so those with weak skills can practice. All of this should be done now before the emergency, but realistically, consider too, in most cases, your plan won't work exactly the way it is supposed to.

For several years I managed a large firearms shop in the Midwest. Each fall literally hundreds of people came

in to buy a new rifle or trade in their old one in antici-
pation of an expensive big game hunting trip. Try as I
might, in all those years I only managed a handful of
times to convince a customer to buy a couple of extra
boxes of ammo so he could learn to handle his new gun
before he got to the field. Most big game hunters get
only one or two chances a season, and usually they blow
the opportunity. Obviously the stakes are higher for the
retreat defender. Perhaps after the collapse and before
the rebuilding starts you can break up the monotony by
working on retreat defense training.

5. Be prepared.
Keep all guns loaded and in convenient locations. If
there is even a remote chance of danger, carry. If you
leave the retreat, the shot you fire may alert the main
crew and save their lives.

Even when my kids were very young, we always
kept loaded guns around the house. They had to learn
that the guns and the damage they could do were real.
Our policy with visiting toddlers was that they had to be
in their parents' control or the family was not welcome.
Usually it was not necessary to say anything because the
parents knew how we lived. Many were so concerned
they never let their kids out of their sight. In a retreat
situation where the living is confined, it will be necessary to control children for other reasons than the presence of loaded guns. But it's a good place to start.

6. Mark your territory.
In Africa, unless we defined exactly at what point
we would open fire with what weapons, the natives
would be so frightened that they would allow themselves to be overrun before starting to fire.
Put marks on the ground, or establish a perimeter

based on things like rocks, bushes, a strand of wire, or a mark on a tree. Timing is extremely important. Be sure that your reaction is not premature or too long in coming. Give this matter some thought and develop a plan based on the realities of your situation.

Marks should also be designated for range determination aids. Weapons sighted in for these predetermined ranges will deliver more accurate, more effective fire.

7. Obscure and camouflage your retreat.

Make it difficult for the enemy to know what their objective should be, why you are fighting, what fighting resources you might have at hand, and where you are firing from.

8. Establish a good, workable command center, along with an alternate if possible.

Go through the numbers with your group so you know that you can actually command from the location you have selected. Be sure you are reasonably protected. Nothing demoralizes a group more than having their leader taken out before the real fighting begins. Be sure to designate a second-in-command, so that if you are hit, the group has another person to guide them out of their predicament.

9. If possible, engage the enemy away from the retreat before they are organized and ready to storm up the hill to your door. This only applies when you are absolutely certain you have no other alternative but to fight.

10. Do not neglect patrolling and guard duty.

These activities are your eyes and ears. They keep you from being surprised. In Africa I had a terrible time keeping our guards awake at night. Finally I started using old women who had had children killed by the raiders and whom I could keep close to me during the day. They had better motivation, and by watching them during the day I could be sure they got some sleep. Of course, these women couldn't shoot, but they could turn on a light and beat on a can if they saw or heard something. It was an effective method of using what few assets I had.

Patrolling and guard duty are especially tough when there is a lot of work to be done around the retreat and everyone is tired and when there is danger outside from NBC agents. In any case you will have to split your people up and use them on a rotational basis. Nobody ever said it would be easy. Just be absolutely sure you don't neglect the chore of looking around on a regular basis.

11. Set up two reaction teams comprised of your best people who can inspire the others to action when the time comes.

Assign the first team the job of forming the main defense. Hold the second team in reserve until you know what you are facing. By establishing a clear set of rehearsed guidelines, you can stimulate people to act. They will know who is to fire at what under what circumstances. You will know when to deploy your fire and explosives and be able to measure their effectiveness.

God be with you. This part of it will not be fun, even if it is interesting.

13. The Ultimate Scenario

THE SURVIVOR WHO PLANS TO fight an organized, trained army is kidding himself. In terms of both materiel and manpower, the cost is far higher than the survivor can afford to pay. There are a few things that can be done to ease the pain, but in general, the survivor had best either flee from the conflict or plan to remain undetected at all costs.

Armies cannot, of course, avoid having to be on the ground where you are in order to destroy you. This is true in spite of modern supersonic jets, helicopter gunships, and artillery with ten-kilometer, pinpoint accuracy. The Nazis found this out in the Warsaw ghetto, for instance. On the other hand, once having decided that your real estate is valuable, organized armies have enormous resources with which to assemble their forces. Troop trucks, armored personnel carriers, and helicopters are good examples.

At times it is possible to keep armies out of your area by lethal harassment that keeps them unsure of exactly where you are or what is happening. An example would be blowing a building down on top of a small patrol. Another would be a couple of blocks of worthless city rubble that you keep clear with well-concealed, intermittent, very accurate sniper fire. If the enemy did send in tanks and helicopters, it would be to occupy some worthless rubble. Most military people make decisions based on rational objectives: if the game isn't worth the candle, they won't play. If your retreat isn't worth the fight, they won't bother you—even if its location is known.

Nevertheless, if tanks and planes are a threat, and you absolutely must protect against them, it sometimes can be done. Just be damn sure it's what you have to do because it's going to be tough, and it's going to be costly. You must evaluate the likelihood of being attacked not only by tanks and planes, but also by artillery, rockets, mortars, heavy machine guns, and in extreme cases, bombers. There is nothing the survivor can do if this is his enemy and the bombardment has started, except to fight as much of a war of attrition as he can. No matter what anybody says, you aren't going to be able to hold out.

During the fighting in Beirut when the PLO was still there, it was their practice to occupy a high-rise office building or apartment complex in the center of town and dynamite the top two or three floors. The rubble on top provided an ideal fire base and also protected the defenders from bombs and artillery. The retreaters themselves occupied several middle floors of the building where they were similarly sheltered. As much as possible, they obstructed the approaches to the buildings against tanks and APCs. The only course open to the attackers was to move up the approaches to the building which were, of course, covered from the upper levels by the defenders. Tanks, RPG-7s, heavy machine guns, rockets, and mortars notwithstanding, the only way the Israelis could take the retreat was to walk in and slug it out with the defenders.

The only weakness to this strategy was resupplying

food, water, and to some extent munitions. You may remember that the Israelis tried to starve out the PLO but
had only limited success. The wily Arabs crept out at
night and bought what they needed from the Lebanese
merchants!

The PLO also dynamited many buildings they didn't
use. Being unsure exactly which buildings to take mate-
rially frustrated the Israeli plan to occupy Beirut, and
the immense amount of rubble the PLO created made
mechanized travel through the narrow streets of the city
that much more difficult.

Lest this experience encourage the survivor to plan
to make war on armies, let me remind you that ulti-
mately the PLO lost, in spite of excellent food and arms
caches, well-developed retreats, and religious zeal.

One alternative is to wage guerrilla war against an
occupying army. As a practical matter for the survivor,
this will not work either. Guerrillas hold no territory.
They have no real retreat and do not really control
events. They maintain some degree of autonomy, but
only at the pleasure of the citizenry and the army
opposing them. In a real survival situation, I doubt that
even guerrillas could operate. Every guerrilla group I
have ever seen required support from a civilian population.

Rural retreaters will have an especially tough time
dealing with organized armies. The only really practical
plan is to destroy bridges and roads and use the natural
terrain such that it isn't worth the invaders' trouble to
attack your retreat. Coupled with some first-rate hiding
techniques so that the soldiers don't know what they
are looking for, the plan might work.

Besides hiding, there really is only one other thing
that the survivor can do now to deal with this situation.
Since large weapons are virtually impossible to acquire,

the next best thing is to assemble a small library on common crew-served weapons. Then maybe you can pick up an RPG-7 or a mortar and use it effectively after the collapse.

I truly wish I had more to offer. Basically, I would urge you not to plan to fight armies, and in so doing not to consider yourself a coward. A retreat is a place to live through the crisis, not a bunker that you as a POW can brag held out for two days instead of two hours.

14. Appendix I — Commercial Sources

By NOW IT SHOULD BE CLEAR that the retreats we are talking about in this book are not log cabins set in pine forests alongside remote, pristine lakes. Retreats, for survivalists, are places that provide shelter from hostile people, elements, and nuclear, biological, and chemical agents. Under some circumstances, a retreat could be both a summer home and a bunker, but for the average survivalist, this is fairly unlikely.

To a large extent, the concept of a defensible bunker and an NBC shelter is a contradiction in terms. A *shelter* must be a buttoned-up, closed-in place that will protect the inhabitants from a chemically hostile environment. A *bunker* is designed primarily to defend strategic locations from hostile intruders. Obviously one cannot defend his bunker if he has his head pulled down so far he doesn't know what is going on outside.

Happily, the solution to all this is not quite as hopeless and contradictory as it might seem. Intruders will not become a problem if your retreat is well hidden, the approaches strong, and the entrance obscured. Secondly, the time of the most intensive biological warfare will not be the time when unwanted visitors will come rambling up to your door.

111

If the collapse occurs as a result of economic failure and mob action is a threat, you will have to rely on the fact that mobs generally have no planned, coordinated goal. You must go out of your way to prevent your retreat from becoming a symbolic target.

Weeks after the collapse, random looters will start to be a problem. Then the answer is regular patrols, listening posts, assigned general guard duty, and your on-the-ground defense net. This is the time to turn your retreat from a shelter to a bunker/command post. Your location and circumstances will determine how far to carry this conversion.

Commercial sources for retreats that combine these two attributes may exist, but I have not seen them. Generally the emphasis is on producing an NBC resistant shelter with no thought at all given to how to defend the place!

Another phenomenon that is even more insidious is the concept of the collective shelter. Virtually every government and commercial publication on shelters and shelter management stresses the desirability of establishing large, group shelters where citizens can gather and withstand the ordeal ahead as a group. One of the first duties of the shelter manager, according to these publications, is to *disarm* the arriving refugees. I sincerely trust that no one who has read this book will ever fall into this kind of trap.

What this boils down to is that probably 95 percent of the time, survivalists will have to modify and harden existing structures in order to turn them into proper retreats. It would be nice to custom build a new house containing an integrated retreat design or to have enough money to call up a contractor and have him put in a professionally designed retreat. But most of the time it doesn't work that way. Most people don't have that kind of money, and commercial plans are scarce. For that reason, I have kept this chapter brief and to the point. It is for the 5 percent who have the dough.

If you are building new, the simplest expedient is to put in an especially heavy, thick-walled basement. You may even want to build an underground home. There are several outfits that have predrawn underground house plans available.

If your local lumberyard doesn't have them, try Underground Homes, Inc., Box 1346, Portsmouth, Ohio 45662. These homes are always touted as being energy efficient. The problem is that energy conservation is no longer fashionable, so there isn't the selection available that there was even a few years ago. Apparently living full-time in a below-ground house is more fun to talk about than to do, a point that the retreater should understand early on.

Some people may want an actual blast shelter. I don't think these are especially necessary unless you live near a missile site. Even people in cities that are likely first-strike targets can develop other, less costly alternatives, assuming they are not absolutely under ground zero. If ground zero is your case, you had better move now or accept your fate. Just remember, ground zero is not nearly as large as the nuclear war hysteria crowd would have you believe. Plans for blast shelters, or if you have enough money, completed structures, are available from Stormaster Shelter Co., 7318 Ferguson Road, Dallas, Texas 75238.

Two firms that make nice prefab fallout shelters are Biosphere Corporation, Box 300, Elk River, Minnesota 55330, and Brodie's Biosphere Corp., Greenfield, New Hampshire 03047. These are basically round batholith-type structures that are delivered complete, ready to place in the hole of your choosing. Along with excavation, there are tremendous added expenses for cement approaches, aprons, stairs, and landscaping that are not included in the purchase price.

The Berryman Shelter Equipment Co., 238 N. Indiana Avenue, Englewood, Florida 33533, has internal equipment and some retreat plans. Don't forget items such as ventilation fans, wood stoves, auxiliary power units, metal shelves, etc., which are commonly available from building supply stores or commercial equipment dealers.

Most commercial architects or engineers are technically competent to design buildings or parts of buildings that will withstand various threat levels. It will be up to you to tell them what you want to guard against. They will design a system and even give you a pretty good idea of what it will cost.

The American Institute of Architects commissioned a national fallout shelter design competition in the late sixties. Many of the winning designs are published in an Office of Civil Defense Technical Report, TR-47, published in July 1967. Most of the work was for large-community school or shopping center complexes. Nevertheless, your architect could take the ideas and incorporate them into your own design. Another publication of the same type gives ideas and plans for smaller buildings. It is *New Buildings with Fallout Protection,* TR-27, 1965, available from the Office of Civil Defense.

Two additional Civil Defense booklets deserve mention because of the excellent general information they contain on hardening techniques for retreats. They are *Interim Guidelines for Building Occupant Protection from Tornadoes and Extreme Winds,* TR-83A and *Increasing Blast and Fire Resistance in Buildings,* TR-62.

It seems to be the fad among survival writers to berate the Civil Defense people for their ancient literature. Personally I find no real problem with the basic concepts and designs developed during the late sixties. Some additional technology has evolved in the area of air filtration, water storage, and food preservation, but these have little to do with basic retreat design. I suggest that you scrounge up these books—some of them are out of print—read them yourself, and decide if you have learned anything.

If you have the bucks to go through with it and are willing to take just a modest amount of time, specing a retreat design is not particularly difficult. Just remember that having spent between $30,000 and $150,000 for the structure, you will also have to stock and man it.

The Swiss have a philosophy about defending their country that applies to expensive, cutsom-built retreats. Yes, they acknowledge, their mountainous country is a fortress. But using a fortress properly requires skill and training. It is no good if it isn't properly manned. That's why every Swiss male between the ages of seventeen and fifty-five does two weeks of active duty every year.

Perhaps I err, but it is my feeling that the average survivor will do better with a retreat that is put together by scrounging rather than one dropped in by a contractor. I can't imagine that more than a handful of survivors will ever elect the route of commercial or prefab retreat construction. Nevertheless, if you decide that's the plan for you, the foregoing information will get you started.

I would appreciate hearing from survivors who have built complete shelters. Items such as size, fixtures, construction techniques, amenities, and cost would be interesting to me.

15. Appendix II—The Defensible Retreat Check List

O<small>NCE</small> YOU HAVE A RETREAT site picked out or are at least evaluating several locations, use a check list to identify your priorities and establish a work plan and a budget. Most of the following points must be answered with a Yes. If there are many answered with a No, either get to work upgrading your retreat or find another location. There is little fluff in the list.

CHECK LIST

Yes or No

___ ___ Will the retreat hold all of the people who are likely to use it?

___ ___ Does the retreat provide inherent protection from nuclear, biological, and chemical threats?

___ ___ Is water available independent of any municipal supply or source?

___ ___ Do I know how I will preserve my food?

— — Have I identified how I will heat and cook?

— — Is it possible to safely store food, clothing, explosives, guns, and ammunition at the retreat?

— — Can the location be secured now before it is actually manned during the collapse?

— — Does it have adequate facilities? Can all these people wash occasionally? Will the toilets work?

— — Can the retreat be obscured and hidden, now and after the fighting starts?

— — Do any neighbors or friends outside of those who will be using the retreat know of its existence?

— — Have I devised a workable defense plan?

— — Can the area be patrolled?

— — Is the retreat actually defensible or am I just kidding myself?

— — Can the approaches be mined and guarded?

— — Do I have the proper equipment to guard them?

___ ___ Is the retreat in an area where I can raise a garden, scrounge, and generally set up a viable existence after the collapse?

___ ___ Do I have a library in the retreat?

___ ___ Is the library good enough to provide the information needed after the collapse? If not, what books do I still need?

___ ___ Do I have adequate amounts of every-thing to implement my mine field and mantrap plans for the retreat, given a fair and honest evaluation of what I will probably have to face?

___ ___ What about medical supplies and infor-mation? Have I got that covered?

___ ___ Have I provided for nuclear/biological monitoring? Do I have Geiger counters, dosimeters, etc.?

___ ___ Do I have decontamination suits so at least some of my people can leave the retreat to guard, patrol, and take care of outside chores?

___ ___ Have I made plans to keep hordes of people from coming anywhere near my area?

___ ___ Have I evaluated my people and at-tempted to fit them into the various duties the best way possible?

—— —— Am I psychologically equipped to defend my retreat? Can I actually shoot intruders?

—— —— Does everyone know which situations will actually trigger the defense plan and when to set off the mines and explosives and start shooting?

—— —— Do I have a stock of barter goods? Are they properly stored?

—— —— Do I know how everyone will get to the retreat? Do they have at least one alternative contingency plan for getting to the retreat, preferably two?

—— —— Have I evaluated the various threat possibilities and then made realistic plans to counter them, especially the nonconfrontive, nonmilitary threats?

—— —— Are the immediate approaches to my retreat such that they can be made impassable by booby traps or just plain physical means?

—— —— Do I know how much time it will take to close the approaches and who will be in charge of this job?

—— —— Do I have a battle plan that fits everyone into the defense structure?

_____ ____ Do I know the warning signs that will indicate that it is time to put my retreat plan into operation?

_____ ____ Do I have the correct guns and enough ammunition or have I been swept away by the armament gurus into believing tons of hardware can replace the right amount of the proper equipment?

_____ ____ Have I planned for retreat communications?

_____ ____ Do I know what means and material the enemy will have at his disposal or even who the enemy is, in a realistic sense?

_____ ____ Have I put together a psychological plan to keep people away and discourage them if they do attack?

_____ ____ Have I planned for special medical/dietary needs of the group?

_____ ____ Have I taken care of my group's current medical/dental requirements so these won't be of immediate concern after the collapse?

_____ ____ Do I know how to handle explosives safely?

_____ ____ . . . reload ammunition?

_____ ____ . . . operate and repair guns?

—— ——   Am I skilled in using alternative means of transportation?

—— ——   Am I highly motivated and self-confident?

—— ——   Do I know my home territory?

—— ——   Have I tried to look at defeating my retreat from the eyes of an enemy?

—— ——   Is the retreat adequately stocked with tools and utensils for use in the new economy?

—— ——   Do I know where to get the consumable items we will need such as light bulbs, grease, oil, toilet paper, soap, canning lids, salt, needles, and thread? Have I thought about these items in terms of my retreat?

—— ——   Are fires a danger? If so, what can I do to counter that threat?

—— ——   Is blast a danger? Will my retreat withstand an explosion?

—— ——   Can I properly evaluate situations? Am I prone to hysteria or passivity?

—— ——   Do I have a continuing survival training program?

—— ——   Have I studied other collapsed societies

and how people are surviving?

— —   Have I made plans to defend against heavy equipment such as tanks and helicopters, if that becomes necessary?

— —   Is it possible for attackers to sneak up on my retreat unseen or, more importantly, for them to detect my retreat without exposing themselves?

— —   Do I know how to use fish, game, and wild plants in my area?

— —   Do I know how to garden in my area?

— —   Do I have a postcollapse skill I can use during the readjustment?

— —   Do I know how the actual retreat will be ventilated? What about lighting?

Obviously this is a check list and not a grocery list. If I were to give you a precise list of things you must do, it would be little better than the government plans. The scheme would not work. Survival is a personal matter. *You* have to work out the exact details of your plan.

16. Bibliography

NUCLEAR SURVIVAL

Clayton, Bruce. *Life After Doomsday*. Boulder, Colorado: Paladin Press, 1981.

Clayton, Mary Ellen and Bruce. *Urban Alert!* Boulder, Colorado: Paladin Press, 1982.

Kearny, Cresson H. *Nuclear War Survival Skills*. Coos Bay, Oregon: NWS Research Bureau, 1980.

Improvised Fallout Shelters in Buildings. Moscow, Idaho: University of Idaho College of Engineering.

Nieman, Thomas. *Better Read Than Dead*. Boulder, Colorado: Paladin Press, 1981.

MEDICAL

Benson, Ragnar. *Survivalist's Medicine Chest*. Boulder, Colorado: Paladin Press, 1982.

Berkow, Robert. *The Merck Manual of Diagnosis and Therapy*. Rahway, New Jersey: Merck & Co. Inc., 1977.

Moore, Marilyn. *Survival Medicine Nature's Way*. Cornville, Arizona: Desert Publications, 1980.

Physicians' Desk Reference. 37th ed. Oradell, New Jersey: Medical Economics Co., 1983.

U.S. Army Special Forces Medical Handbook. Boulder, Colorado: Paladin Press, 1982.

GUNS AND AMMUNITION

Givens, Tom. *Survival Shooting.* Cornville, Arizona: Desert Publications, 1980.

Shaw, John and Bane, Michael. *You Can't Miss, The Guide to Combat Pistol Shooting.* Memphis, Tennessee: Mid-South Institute of Self Defense, 1982.

Tappan, Melrose. *Survival Guns.* The Janus Press: Rogue River, Oregon, 1980.

Taylor, Chuck. *The Complete Book of Combat Handgunning.* Cornville, Arizona: Desert Publications, 1982.

EXPLOSIVES

Improvised Munitions/Black Books Volumes 1 and 2. Boulder, Colorado: Paladin Press, 1980.

OSS Sabotage and Demolition Manual. Boulder, Colorado: Paladin Press, 1980.

Powell, William. *The Anarchist Cookbook.* Lyle Stuart Inc., Secaucus, New Jersey, 1971.

The Chemistry of Powder and Explosives. Boulder, Colorado: Paladin Press, 1979.

LIVING OFF THE LAND

Benson, Ragnar. *Eating Cheap.* Boulder, Colorado: Paladin Press, 1982.

Benson, Ragnar. *Live Off the Land in the City and Country.* Boulder, Colorado: Paladin Press, 1981.

Benson, Ragnar. *Survival Poaching.* Boulder, Colorado: Paladin Press, 1980.

Casey, Douglas R., *Crisis Investing.* Atlanta, Georgia: '76 Press, 1979.

Stoner, Carol Hupping. *Stocking Up.* Emmaus, Pennsylvania: Rodale Press, 1977.

BOOBY TRAPS

Benson, Ragnar. *Mantrapping.* Boulder, Colorado: Paladin Press, 1980.
Booby Traps. Boulder, Colorado: Paladin Press. 1978.

TACTICS

Idreiss, Ion L. *The Scout.* Boulder, Colorado: Paladin Press, 1978.
Ranger Handbook. Boulder, Colorado: Paladin Press, 1978.
Special Forces Operational Techniques. Boulder, Colorado: Paladin Press, 1979.
Special Forces Reconnaissance Handbook. Boulder, Colorado: Paladin Press, 1980.
Levy, Bert "Yank", *Guerrilla Warfare.* Boulder, Colorado: Paladin Press, 1979.

THE OFFICE OF CIVIL DEFENSE

Aboveground Home Shelters
Family Home Shelter Designs (PSD F-61-1)
Home Shelter (H-12-1)
Increasing Blast and Fire Resistance in Buildings, TR-62
Interim Guidelines for Building Occupant Protection from Tornadoes and Extreme Winds, TR-83A
Office of Civil Defense Technical Report, TR-47
New Buildings with Fallout Protection, TR-27

PSYCHOLOGY

Brown, Mark H. *The Flight of the Nez Percé.*   Lincoln, Nebraska: University of Nebraska Press, 1974.
Solzhenitsyn, Aleksandr. *The Gulag Archipelago.* New York: Harper and Row, 1979.